Prolapse Exercises

Inside Out

A Complete Guide to
Prolapse Exercises
for Women

Michelle Kenway
Pelvic Floor Physiotherapist

Prolapse Exercises Inside Out

A Complete Guide to Prolapse Exercises for Women

www.pelvicexercises.com.au

Published by Healthy Fit Solutions Pty Ltd

ISBN 978-0-6469045-7-3

Photography: Mike Curtin

Illustrations: Ryan McDonald-Smith

Editing: Tania Paul

Contents

Introduction

"A chain is only as strong as its weakest link"

Proverb

The weakest link for many women with prolapse is their pelvic floor.

Prolapse can affect much more than a woman's pelvic floor - prolapse problems frequently affect a woman's ability or perceived ability to exercise. Women are usually concerned, and at times quite terrified about general exercises worsening their prolapse or causing repeat prolapse having already undergone prolapse surgery. For women with coexisting health problems such as osteoporosis or weight management problems, the whole issue of how to exercise with a prolapse can become confusing and disheartening. As a direct result, many women needlessly cease exercise altogether, and in doing so, forgo the wonderful benefits exercise provides for their long-term physical and psychological health and wellbeing.

Many women with prolapse can continue to exercise safely and effectively by improving their pelvic floor support and adopting 'pelvic floor safe exercise' - the phrase and concept first introduced in Inside Out, the foundation book in this series.

Unfortunately there is no one rule for all women seeking to exercise safely with prolapse problems. Women differ with respect to the capacity of their pelvic floor to support general exercises as well as individual risk factors that may increase their likelihood of prolapse problems with inappropriate exercises. For example some women with prolapse and well functioning pelvic floor supports may be able to exercise at a more intense and varied level than other women with poor pelvic floor support and/or severe or recurrent prolapse problems. The general pelvic floor safe exercise principles outlined in this book emphasize low impact fitness exercises, appropriate core abdominal training and modified strength training and these principles will usually apply to most women with prolapse problems.

There are 3 key areas of understanding outlined in this book to help you exercise:

- How to maximise your pelvic organ (and prolapse) support.
- How to avoid those exercises with potential to overload the pelvic floor.
- How to choose the most appropriate and effective pelvic floor safe exercises for your exercise needs.

Prolapse Exercises is divided into three exercise sections.

Section 1 helps you better understand your prolapse and how to improve your pelvic floor support for general exercise.

Section 2 shows you how to identify and choose appropriate exercises for your body, with pelvic floor safe exercise guidance for prolapse and muscle strength training, core abdominal and general fitness exercises.

Section 3 assists women with special exercise recovery needs before and after prolapse repair surgery, exercises for osteoporosis and guidance for prolapse and weight management exercise.

I am delighted to bring you Prolapse Exercises the follow-on to Inside Out. I sincerely hope that this information gives you the tools you need to exercise with confidence, achieve your health and fitness goals and enjoy an active life.

Michelle Kenway

Prolapse Exercises FAQ

A number of frequently asked questions have emerged in relation to safe exercise with a prolapse and many of these are listed here to provide you with an overview to the content of Prolapse Exercises. The answers to these types of frequently asked questions are expanded upon in the subsequent chapters of this book.

I've been diagnosed with a prolapse. Can I continue to exercise?

Many women become unnecessarily alarmed about their ability to exercise with a prolapse - for most women exercise is desirable and should be encouraged. Unless you've been advised otherwise by your doctor, being diagnosed with a prolapse is usually no reason to cease general exercise altogether. Muscle strength and endurance exercises may in fact help to reduce the overall pressure on your pelvic floor and prolapse during your everyday activities. The key to safe exercise with prolapse problems is to adopt pelvic floor safe exercises and techniques long-term.

Will pelvic floor exercises reverse my prolapse?

Pelvic floor exercises can't reverse a prolapse. A pelvic prolapse is a defect (like a hernia) in the vaginal walls and strong supporting tissues that support the internal pelvic organs. Pelvic floor exercise can't reverse these overstretched tissues once stretched. In some cases pelvic floor exercises can, however, decrease prolapse symptoms as well as lift the pelvic floor (and prolapse) to sit higher within the pelvis.

Can pelvic floor exercises reduce the likelihood of repeat prolapse after my surgery?

Women have everything to gain from improving pelvic floor support prior to and following prolapse surgery. Effective pelvic floor exercises may reduce the likelihood of repeat prolapse after prolapse surgery as well as reduce the likelihood of associated bladder or bowel problems, especially if your pelvic floor muscles are weak.

Will pelvic floor exercises improve my prolapse symptoms?

Yes, for some women with intact pelvic floor muscles and mild to moderately severe prolapse, pelvic floor exercises can improve prolapse symptoms. Pelvic floor exercises are unlikely to improve prolapse symptoms in women who have had serious pelvic floor nerve or muscle tearing (avulsion) injury, and/or women with severe prolapse.

Can pelvic floor exercises prevent my prolapse from becoming worse?

If your pelvic floor muscles are weak or not working as they should, effective pelvic floor exercises may improve internal support for your prolapsed organs. Pelvic floor exercises should be incorporated as part of a whole body prolapse management approach, along with modification of known risk factors for prolapse such as poor bowel emptying patterns and excess body weight.

Will my prolapse become worse if I exercise?

For many women, pelvic floor safe exercises will allow them to exercise without worsening their prolapse or exacerbating their prolapse symptoms. The exercises you can perform are ultimately determined by many factors, including how well your pelvic floor is supporting your prolapse and the severity of your prolapse. If your pelvic floor muscles aren't working well, inappropriate exercises and/or techniques may contribute to worsening prolapse symptoms. Women who have well functioning pelvic floor muscles and prolapse may find that they can perform a wide variety of exercise and remain untroubled by prolapse symptoms or worsening prolapse severity.

When can I return to general exercise after prolapse surgery?

Your gynaecologist will advise you when it's safe for you to return to exercise after your prolapse repair surgery. Your doctor's decision will be based upon factors including the surgical procedure used, post-operative problems, your overall recovery and individual risk of repeat prolapse. When you have your doctor's approval to return to exercise, your pelvic floor safe exercise program should be gradually progressed over time to help reduce your risk of repeat prolapse. It is often inappropriate for women to return directly to their previous exercise program after prolapse surgery.

I have had prolapse surgery in the past, how much weight can I safely lift?

Your gynaecologist may set an upper limit on how much you can lift - always be guided by this limit. Many factors potentially influence how much weight you can safely lift: the height from which you lift, your physical strength, the load placed on your pelvic floor by your abdominal body fat and your pelvic organ support (pelvic floor muscle strength and size of your vagina). Furthermore, different muscle groups in a woman's body usually vary in strength so that there is no one weight appropriate for different resistance exercises. It is vital that you never lift or attempt to move any load that makes you strain.

I've been diagnosed with a prolapse. How can I manage my body weight if I need to avoid high impact exercise?

Women often fear that changing their exercise program to manage their prolapse will cause them to gain weight. A prolapse diagnosis doesn't mean you're going to gain weight. A combination of sensible diet and pelvic floor safe exercise is most desirable to manage body weight.

To control your body weight, manage your energy intake (food and drink) as a priority. It takes a lot of exercise to burn up excess kilojoules, particularly if your energy intake is very high. The most essential step to avoiding weight gain is to ensure that your diet is controlled and appropriate for your needs. Speak with a qualified dietician for dietary advice if you need help to manage your diet and avoid weight gain.

Pelvic floor safe exercises will also help you manage your body weight and protect your pelvic floor. If you are overweight, losing weight can help you reduce the load on your pelvic floor during general upright exercise. Moderate intensity, low impact fitness exercises, such as cycling or brisk walking, can help you burn energy and lose weight. Pelvic floor safe strength training exercises will help you stay in shape by building lean muscle, toning your body and helping you stay active.

I was diagnosed with a prolapse 3 weeks after the birth of my second child. How can I return to exercise to help me lose weight I gained during pregnancy?

Exercise with prolapse after childbirth presents a new mum with some unique challenges. Weight gained during pregnancy increases the load on the pelvic floor. Hormonal changes with breast feeding and increased fatigue can prolong the time taken to recover pelvic floor strength and support. New mums can usually undertake progressive low impact moderate intensity exercises such as brisk walking or stationary cycling when the pelvic floor is sufficiently healed. Pelvic floor safe light resistance training and deep abdominal core control exercises also help women strengthen, tone and improve their ability to cope with the physical demands of motherhood.

Prolapse management exercise after childbirth includes restoring pelvic floor muscle support with progressive pelvic floor exercises. After childbirth, some women with prolapse find that a support pessary can help them to cope with the physical demands of caring for their baby and exercise, while they recover their pelvic floor strength and support.

Why shouldn't I run after prolapse surgery? All my friends are still running - even with prolapse problems

Running is a high impact exercise and high impact exercises have potential to overload the weak pelvic floor, especially when repeated over time. If you've ever noticed bladder leakage with jumping or stepping heavily, you will know first-hand the effect of impact and associated pressure upon your pelvic floor. Running creates repeated impact on the pelvic floor which causes already weakened pelvic organ supports to progressively stretch and further weaken over time.

After prolapse surgery most women should avoid high impact exercises. Unfortunately some women undergo prolapse repair with the misguided intention of returning to running. If you have a prolapse and your pelvic floor muscles are not working well, low impact fitness exercises are the safest alternative for the long-term protection of your pelvic floor repair. Stationary cycling is one form of exercise that can give you a great fitness workout without compromising your pelvic floor.

I've been diagnosed with osteoporosis and I've been advised to do strength exercises. I had a prolapse repair a few years ago - can I go to the gym?

Gym-based strength training exercises are often prescribed for women with decreased bone density. Strength training exercises for osteoporosis aim to load the bones with unusual strain. When bones are appropriately loaded and placed under unusual strain, the bone responds with a signal to produce new bone cells. Loading bones is typically achieved by lifting heavy weights, however heavy weight loaded exercises are not appropriate for women with prolapse related problems, especially after prolapse surgery. If you go to the gym, you will require a modified pelvic floor safe strength training program for your bone health.

Modified strength training for bone health and prolapse needs to be an individually prescribed pelvic floor safe program rather than a one-fits-all strength training program. Bone loading for bone health can be promoted through exercises other than heavy resistance exercises. There are a range of exercises that can be performed to help load those areas of the body at-risk of fracture without lifting heavy weights or compromising the pelvic floor. Some pelvic floor safe resistance exercises can be loaded to promote improved bone health.

Are spin classes safe with a prolapse?

Spin classes are stationary cycle classes offered in many fitness centres. Spin classes usually include alternating high and low levels of pedal resistance, along with alternating cycle speeds. Stationary cycling is low impact exercise and therefore a pelvic floor safe form of aerobic fitness and weight control exercise for most women with mild to moderate prolapse. To keep spin classes pelvic floor safe:

- Use low to moderate resistance when pedalling and always avoid straining with high resistance through your legs.
- Stay seated in the bike seat throughout the class - avoid standing out of the saddle and using high gears during climbing tracks.

I've read that I should avoid sit ups (abdominal curls) with my prolapse. How can I exercise for a flatter stomach?

One of the biggest myths about abdominal exercise is that sit up exercises flatten the stomach. Sit up exercises can't reduce abdominal fat. Intense abdominal curl exercises (sit ups) increase the downward pressure on the pelvic floor and are inappropriate abdominal exercises for women with prolapse and poorly functioning pelvic floor muscles. Mature women naturally store body weight around their abdomen and those women with visible abdominal 'six-pack' muscles are usually have very low levels of body fat.

A twofold approach can help tone and flatten the general appearance of the lower abdomen. Overall weight loss is the first step which can be achieved by undertaking whole body aerobic fitness exercises and diet modification. Deep abdominal core exercises will also help tone the lower abdomen and these types of exercise can be readily incorporated into pelvic floor safe exercise programs.

Can I squat safely with a prolapse?

Squats are great thigh and buttock strengthening exercises for women. Wide leg deep squats that involve bending forwards from the hips, swinging a kettle bell between the legs or lifting weights from ground level, increase the pressure on the pelvic floor supports. Pressure on the pelvic floor increases with heavily weighted, deep squats. Pelvic floor safe squats involve using appropriate loads that avoid strain and keeping squats shallow rather than deep. Mini squats and exercise ball to wall squats are pelvic floor safe alternatives to the deep wide leg squats common place in fitness centres.

Is Pilates the right choice of exercise with a prolapse?

Pilates exercise incorporates core abdominal exercises originally designed for spinal support and control. Some women with or at risk of pelvic floor problems commence Pilates and find that they develop or worsen their existing pelvic floor symptoms. There are some Pilates exercises that are appropriate and pelvic floor safe, while the more intense Pilates floor and machine-based core abdominal resistance exercises are not appropriate for women with prolapse and pelvic floor muscle dysfunction.

Pelvic floor safe Pilates exercises take into account a woman's pelvic floor risk factors, her prolapse severity and how well her pelvic floor is providing internal support. Intense core abdominal Pilates exercises can often be modified to avoid pelvic floor overload in women with, or at risk of prolapse problems. Women with prolapse also need to be taught how to relax their pelvic floor muscles back to normal resting level having once contracted them during Pilates exercises. Pilates exercises for women who have had previous prolapse surgery need to be carefully prescribed and approached with caution.

Is Yoga pelvic floor safe with a prolapse?

Some Yoga poses have the potential to impact upon the pelvic floor, while others are considered pelvic floor safe. The risk posed by Yoga to a woman's pelvic floor depends on many factors: the Yoga poses, instructor techniques, level of ability of the class, individual pelvic floor function and capacity to withstand the pressure associated with different Yoga poses.

In general terms, pelvic floor safe Yoga poses:

- Avoid intense abdominal muscle bracing
- Avoid breath holding and straining
- Avoid sustained and intense core abdominal contraction
- Minimise the amount of body weight supported through the upper limbs
- Avoid wide leg deep squats
- Avoid wide leg forward bends
- Promote appropriate contraction and relaxation of pelvic floor muscles.

Most importantly, pelvic floor safe Yoga poses are matched to a woman's pelvic floor capacity - women with poorly functioning pelvic floor muscles and those with pelvic organ prolapse problems will benefit by adopting pelvic floor safe Yoga practice.

I attend a ladies fitness centre, are my circuit class exercises pelvic floor safe?

Unfortunately you can't assume that just because you attend a women's fitness centre the exercises and equipment are pelvic floor safe. While sometimes the size of exercise equipment is better suited to women, the risks to your pelvic floor are similar to those posed by some of the same exercises and equipment found in regular gyms and fitness centres. In particular, women with prolapse need to be mindful of circuit equipment likely to increase the load on the pelvic floor such as resisted leg press, resisted abdominal strength exercises and weight loaded squats.

You will have an immediate understanding of how well your fitness centre classes cater to women with pelvic floor problems by the type of pre-exercise screening that is administered when you first attend. Pre-exercise screening helps to identify women who are at risk of pelvic floor problems and is usually in the form of a pre-exercise questionnaire. Does the pre-exercise questionnaire include some questions to assess your pelvic floor risk factors? If there is no pelvic floor safe exercise program in place, you may benefit from speaking with your instructor about modifying your exercise program if you feel this is feasible.

Can I do Zumba classes after prolapse repair surgery?

Dance classes such as Zumba are usually low impact and therefore pelvic floor safe exercise classes for women. After prolapse repair, your pelvic floor is at increased risk of injury. Be mindful of the potential for Zumba classes to vary from one instructor to the next and remain alert for the need to modify high impact (both feet off the ground) exercises to lower impact exercises. If any Zumba exercises involve jumping or hopping, you can usually reduce the impact by substituting low impact exercises such as side steps or forward steps so that one foot stays on the ground as you exercise.

Section 1

Pelvic Support Exercises

1 Understanding Your Prolapse

What is a Pelvic Organ Prolapse?

A pelvic organ prolapse is like a hernia where supporting tissues in the pelvis are unable to hold the pelvic organs in the correct position. Your pelvic organs include your bladder, vagina, uterus and rectum.

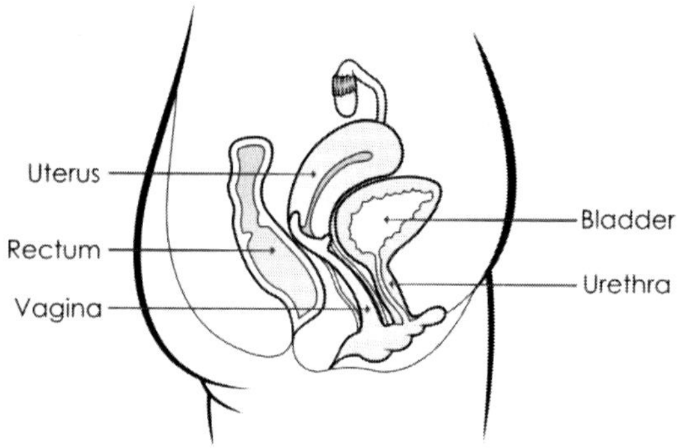

Pelvic organs side view

The pelvic organs are held in their correct position by the pelvic floor muscles and tissues within the pelvis. When these pelvic supports are strained, they can stretch and weaken so that they become unable to retain the pelvic organs in their correct position. As a result, one or more of the pelvic organs can move down into the vagina and this is known as a pelvic organ prolapse.

Types of Pelvic Organ Prolapse

There are different types of pelvic organ prolapse, some occur more commonly than others.

Anterior vaginal wall prolapse (bladder prolapse or cystocoele)

Bladder prolapse is one of the most commonly occurring forms of pelvic prolapse. A bladder prolapse occurs when the bladder moves into the front (or anterior) wall of the vagina. This happens when the bladder moves backward into the front wall of the vagina. When a bladder prolapse is severe the front wall of the vagina may bulge out of and become visible at the vaginal opening.

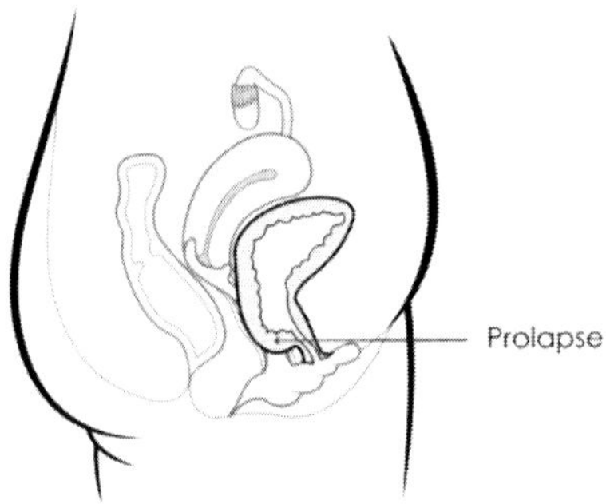

Cystocoele side view

Posterior vaginal wall prolapse (rectocoele)

When the lower part of the bowel (rectum) moves forward into the back wall of the vagina, this is known as posterior vaginal wall prolapse. This type of prolapse may be visible as a bulge at the opening of the vagina when more severe and often becomes more noticeable after a bowel movement or with straining to empty the bowels. This type of bowel prolapse into the vagina is not the same as a rectal prolapse described further in this chapter.

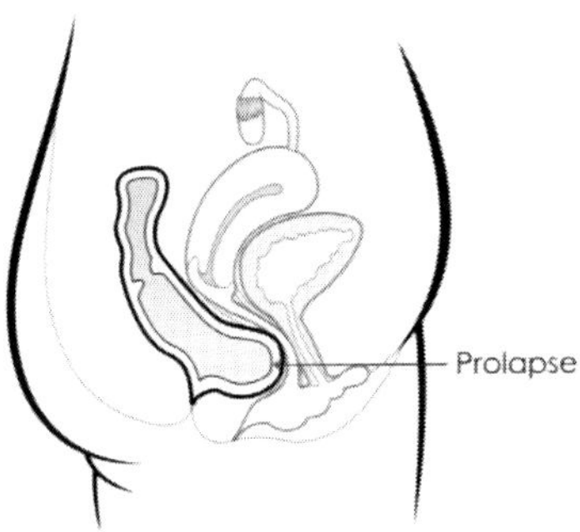

Rectocoele side view

Uterine prolapse

Uterine prolapse occurs when the uterus (womb) and cervix descend into the vagina from the normal position above the vagina. In women who have had a hysterectomy, the upper part of the vagina can move down within the vagina and this is known as a vaginal vault prolapse.

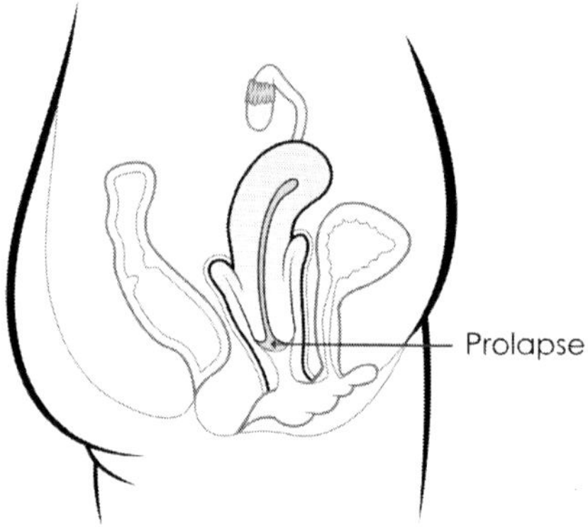

Uterine prolapse side view

Symptoms of Pelvic Organ Prolapse

Prolapse symptoms can vary among women and don't always correspond directly with prolapse severity. Some women are completely unaware of any prolapse symptoms and may not realise they have a prolapse. Prolapse symptoms are usually worse with prolonged upright positions (e.g. standing) and relieved with lying down.

Symptoms of pelvic organ prolapse include:

- Vaginal bulging
- Pelvic heaviness or pressure
- Lower back ache
- Lower abdominal pressure or discomfort
- Bladder emptying problems
- Bowel emptying problems
- Needing to manually reposition the prolapse to empty the bladder or bowel.

What Causes Pelvic Organ Prolapse?

A pelvic prolapse results from weakness in the pelvic floor support structures. When the pelvic floor muscles are weak or damaged, pelvic floor support is decreased and added load is placed upon the strong ligaments and tissues that hold the pelvic organs in the correct position. When this support system is overloaded the pelvic muscles and tissues stretch and weaken allowing the pelvic organs to move downwards into the vagina resulting in pelvic organ prolapse.

What are the Risk Factors for Prolapse?

Some of the risk factors for prolapse in women are an unavoidable part of life. There are a number of known risk factors that may be managed to help reduce the risk of prolapse or repeat prolapse after prolapse surgery. If you have a prolapse, or if you are seeking to avoid repeat prolapse, being aware of prolapse risk factors and managing your controllable risks may help you reduce your risk of repeat prolapse or prolapse worsening. Assess your prolapse risk and take the Prolapse Quiz (p 109).

Pelvic organ prolapse risk factors include:

- Pregnancy and childbirth
- Menopause and increasing age
- Obesity and being overweight (body mass index >25)*
- Chronic constipation and straining*
- Previous pelvic surgery (including prolapse surgery)
- Pelvic floor muscle dysfunction*
- Regular heavy lifting*
- Exercise overload*

*Risk factors for prolapse that may be managed in some women

What is the Long-Term Prognosis for Prolapse?

Left untreated a pelvic organ prolapse will not heal or disappear on its own accord. A prolapse involves pelvic tissues being stretched beyond their normal limits. Once overstretched, the tissues cannot return to their former length. Prolapse seems to worsen with increasing age however this doesn't apply to all women. Some women will have no change in their prolapse for many years, while others find that their prolapse rapidly worsens from a mild prolapse to a more severe condition. Some mild to moderate prolapse conditions can improve with pelvic floor rehabilitation (Chapter 2).

Pelvic Organ Prolapse Severity

Your gynaecologist or pelvic floor physiotherapist will usually assess your prolapse severity. You may be informed that you have a mild, moderate or severe prolapse according to your symptoms and the amount of downward movement of your prolapse evident during examination.

Prolapse severity is usually measured in stages according to an international system of measurement called the POP-Q.[1] This system measures the amount of downward movement of landmarks within the vagina and does not take into account your prolapse symptoms - it classifies prolapse severity according to measurement. The stages of prolapse severity may be graded from Stage 0 (no prolapse demonstrated) to Stage IV (complete eversion or outward movement of the lower genital tract).

Rectal Prolapse

Rectal prolapse is a condition distinct from but often confused with pelvic organ prolapse. Rectal prolapse involves the rectum, not the vagina. The confusion often arises from the fact that the bowel can prolapse into the vagina as in the case of posterior vaginal wall

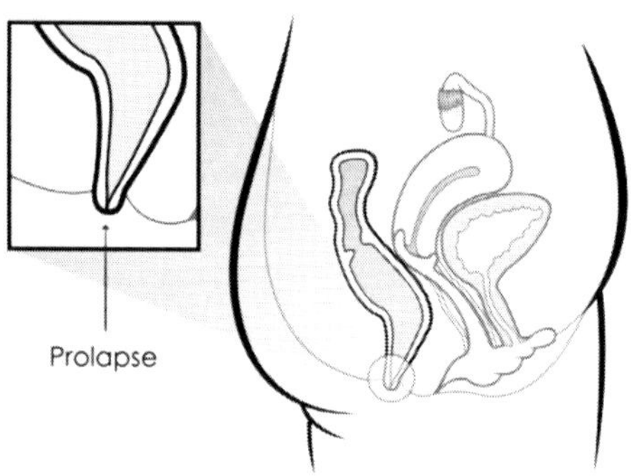

Rectal prolapse side view

prolapse (rectocoele), or it can prolapse within the rectum (rectal prolapse).

Rectal prolapse is included in this book since pelvic floor exercises for support and pelvic floor safe exercise principles also apply to women seeking to manage and exercise with a rectal prolapse or after rectal prolapse surgery.

What is a Rectal Prolapse?

A rectal prolapse involves the lower part of the bowel or rectum moving out of position downwards towards the anus, and sometimes protruding out of the anus.

There are three types of rectal prolapse:

- *Mucosal prolapse* (or partial prolapse) involves only the membrane lining the rectum, known as the rectal mucosa protruding through the anus.
- *Full thickness rectal prolapse* (or complete rectal prolapse) where the rectal wall slides out of place and protrudes through the anus.
- *Internal intussusception* where part of the bowel collapses and slides over itself, but stays inside the body and does not protrude from the anus. The following information does not apply to internal intussuseption.

What Causes Rectal Prolapse?

A rectal prolapse results when the supportive tissues that hold the rectum in position become weakened. A rectal prolapse usually develops as a result of pelvic floor muscle weakness, anal sphincter weakness and looseness (laxity) of the rectal tissues.

Signs and Symptoms of Rectal Prolapse

Some rectal prolapse symptoms are directly associated with the prolapse, while others can develop indirectly owing to the associated difficulties with cleanliness and hygiene.

Signs and symptoms of rectal prolapse include:

- A bulge or protrusion of red coloured tissue from the anus which may be visible especially after a bowel movement
- Staining of underwear and faecal incontinence
- Sensation of wetness and mucous discharge
- Constipation, straining and needing to manually assist bowel emptying
- Sensation of incomplete bowel emptying
- General discomfort around the anus often worse after activity and towards the end of the day

With worsening of rectal prolapse, the associated symptoms usually become more apparent. When less severe, a rectal prolapse will usually retract (move back inside the anus) after a bowel movement. As the prolapse worsens, it protrudes more readily with increased pressure during activities such as heavy lifting, coughing and sneezing. Severe rectal prolapse becomes evident with standing and walking. When the rectal prolapse protrudes from the anus and cannot be repositioned inside the anus this is a medical emergency.

Risk Factors for Rectal Prolapse

- Pelvic floor muscle dysfunction
- Chronic constipation and straining
- Chronic diarrhoea
- Pelvic floor tissue damage during childbirth
- Nerve damage affecting the pelvic floor
- Previous anal surgery
- Heavy lifting
- Ageing

Key Points for Understanding Your Prolapse

- A pelvic organ prolapse is a condition where one or more pelvic organs moves downward into the vagina.
- A pelvic organ prolapse occurs when the supporting tissues in the pelvis are unable to retain the pelvic organs in their normal position.
- Supports for the pelvic organs include pelvic floor muscles and strong pelvic tissues.
- Commonly occurring forms of pelvic organ prolapse involve the bladder, bowel and/or uterus.
- Managing modifiable prolapse risk factors may reduce the risk of repeat prolapse after prolapse surgery.
- Modifiable risk factors for prolapse include regular heavy lifting, exercise overload, constipation and straining, pelvic floor dysfunction, and being overweight.
- Prolapse symptoms vary from woman to woman and don't always correspond with prolapse severity.
- The rate of prolapse progression is unknown and differs from woman to woman.
- Untreated pelvic organ prolapse will not heal.
- Pelvic floor muscle training may reduce prolapse severity and prolapse symptoms in some women.
- Rectal prolapse is a different condition to posterior vaginal wall prolapse (rectocoele).
- Rectal prolapse symptoms usually become more apparent as the prolapse worsens.

2 Exercises for Prolapse Support

Improving the condition of your pelvic floor with regular pelvic floor exercise is a positive step you can take towards improving support for your prolapse, preventing repeat prolapse and staying active long-term.

Pelvic Floor Exercises for Prolapse Support

Pelvic floor exercises (Kegels) can help you manage and even improve some prolapse problems. Women with pelvic floor prolapse are known to have decreased pelvic floor muscle strength.[2] Supervised pelvic floor muscle training has been shown to decrease prolapse symptoms[3] while in some women with mild to moderately severe prolapse, pelvic floor rehabilitation including pelvic floor exercises decreases prolapse severity.[4]

How can Pelvic Floor Muscle Training Help?

Pelvic floor muscle training may assist prolapse management by:

1. Improving pelvic floor strength and pelvic organ support so your pelvic floor can withstand increased pressure during everyday activities and exercises.
2. Teaching how to contract your pelvic floor muscles to prevent downwards movement of your pelvic organs before and during episodes of increased pressure using a technique called 'The Knack'.[5]

Pelvic Floor Rehabilitation and Prolapse Surgery

Pelvic floor muscle training may assist in long-term management after prolapse surgery, however this remains to be confirmed by scientific studies. In women who have undergone previous prolapse surgery the risk of repeat prolapse is increased.[6] It is currently recommended that women undergoing pelvic organ prolapse surgery receive specialised pelvic floor rehabilitation to improve long term support for the prolapse repair and reduce the likelihood of repeat prolapse or new pelvic floor problems developing after surgery.[5]

Prolapse repair surgery aims to restore passive support for the pelvic organs. The active supports for the pelvic organs are the pelvic floor muscles. Pelvic floor exercises can help you ensure that your pelvic floor muscles are in their best possible condition, so that your active and passive supports are working to support your pelvic organs after surgery.

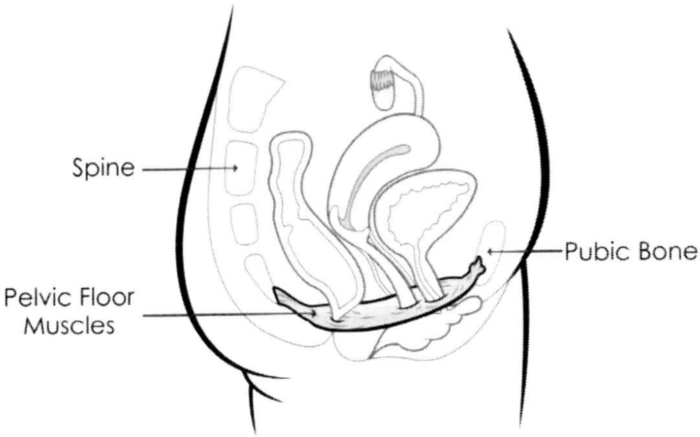

Pelvic Floor

How to Find Your Pelvic Floor Muscles with a Prolapse?

The first step to finding your pelvic floor muscles is to understand where they are located within your body. Your pelvic floor muscles are positioned in layers, in and around the area where you sit, known as the base of your pelvis. They are like a mini trampoline, designed to actively support your pelvic organs and in doing so help prevent prolapse. Your pelvic floor muscles sling front to back from your pubic bone to your tail bone and side to side between the bones you sit on. These muscles also encircle your pelvic openings (urine tube, vagina and anus) as shown on previous page.

Correct Pelvic Floor Muscle Contraction

It is very important that you can feel your pelvic floor muscles contracting using the correct action. Performing the wrong technique by bulging or straining your pelvic floor downwards can potentially worsen your prolapse symptoms. If you're unsure, seek the assistance of a pelvic floor physiotherapist to teach you the correct action for your pelvic floor exercises.

Correct pelvic floor exercise for all types of prolapse involves lifting inwards and squeezing in and around your three pelvic openings - urethra (urine tube), vagina and anus, then relaxing your pelvic floor muscles back to resting position.

Simple Steps to Feel Your Pelvic Floor Muscles

These simple steps are designed to help you find and feel your pelvic floor muscles around your three pelvic openings. Sometimes it can be difficult to feel your pelvic floor muscles contracting, especially if they are weak. Your ability to feel your pelvic floor muscles working can improve as your pelvic floor muscles strengthen and recover. It's important that you can feel the correct exercise technique before commencing your regular pelvic floor workout otherwise you might practice the wrong technique.

Step1

Imagine stopping or slowing the flow of urine having once started - lift and squeeze the muscles in and around the opening to your urine tube. Only do this as an occasional test of your pelvic floor muscles not as a regular exercise and never if you have difficulty emptying your bladder.

Step 2

Imagine lifting and squeezing the muscles in and around your vagina as if to resist withdrawing a tampon.

Step 3

Imagine you need to avoid passing wind (gas) in public by lifting and squeezing the muscles in and around your anus.

Step 4

Combine these 3 steps - lifting and squeezing in and around all three pelvic openings at once. Try to keep lifting and squeezing your pelvic floor muscles and continue to breathe normally. Then completely relax your pelvic floor muscles back to resting.

Tips for Pelvic Floor Exercises and Prolapse

These tips can help you exercise your pelvic floor muscles with a prolapse:

- Practice your pelvic floor exercises early in your day - this is when your pelvic floor muscles will work most effectively and your prolapse is least likely to bulge and weigh down your pelvic floor.
- When starting out you may find your exercises easier to do lying down rather than standing up. The load on your pelvic floor is decreased when lying down which may help you exercise if your pelvic floor is weak.
- If you notice your prolapse bulging down during your exercises, you may be using the wrong exercise technique. Cease your pelvic floor exercises and seek professional assistance to ensure your technique is correct.

- You may consider using a support pessary to assist with your prolapse management as this can sometimes improve the ease of pelvic floor exercises with a prolapse. A support pessary is a device that is inserted into the vagina to lift prolapsed tissues. Speak with your gynaecologist about your suitability for using a pessary if you are considering this management option.

Daily Pelvic Floor Exercise Routine

When you can perform the correct pelvic floor exercise technique, you are ready to commence your regular pelvic floor exercise routine.

To strengthen your pelvic floor muscles aim to:

- Complete up to 8-12 pelvic floor exercises in a row.
- Maintain each exercise for up to 10 seconds, lifting and squeezing your pelvic floor muscles throughout.
- Relax your pelvic floor muscles after every contraction.
- Rest your pelvic floor muscles until recovered between every exercise.
- Perform 10 successive brisk 1-2 second pelvic floor exercises.
- Complete 3 sets of daily pelvic floor exercises.

Progressing Your Exercises

You will need to progress your pelvic floor exercises to make your pelvic floor muscles stronger.

When starting out

Start with the number of pelvic floor exercises you can comfortably manage - everyone is different. Your initial focus should be on contracting your pelvic floor muscles using the correct technique, just like learning a new strength exercise in the gym.

Number of exercises

When starting out you may find you can only perform a few pelvic floor exercises in a row. This is a common experience with weak pelvic floor muscles. Your goal is to gradually build up the number of exercises you can repeat in succession.

Duration of exercises

It may not be possible to maintain each exercise for 10 seconds when you commence training. Start by contracting your pelvic floor muscles for as long as you can with every exercise. With practice you should find that you can maintain each exercise for longer.

Rest breaks

There is no set rule for how long to rest your pelvic floor muscles between exercises. When starting out your pelvic floor muscles will need longer to rest and recover between every effort, 30-45 seconds rest is quite acceptable. As your pelvic floor condition improves, try to reduce the time spent resting your pelvic floor before your next effort.

Position changes

Upright training positions will improve the ability of your pelvic floor muscles to support your pelvic organs during your everyday activities. Exercising your pelvic floor in upright positions trains your pelvic floor muscles to work against the load of your abdomen combined with gravity. When starting out you may need to do your exercises lying down to reduce the load on your pelvic floor. Some women find that they can do their morning exercises sitting or standing and then later in the day when their pelvic floor is fatigued they exercise lying down. Ultimately try to complete all your pelvic floor exercises in upright positions.

Common Mistakes to Avoid

Using the wrong exercise technique can worsen prolapse symptoms or make you think that you are exercising your pelvic floor muscles when in fact you are not.

Common mistakes with pelvic floor exercises include:

- Bearing down
- Breath holding
- Squeezing the inner thighs and buttocks
- Strongly contracting the upper abdominal muscles
- Doing too many pelvic floor exercises - advice to perform hundreds of daily pelvic floor exercises is not consistent with the current principles of muscle strength training and can overfatigue pelvic floor muscles making prolapse symptoms worse

How Long Before You Notice Results?

The length of time required for your pelvic floor training to show an effect depends on a number of factors including:

- The condition of your pelvic floor muscles at the outset
- How much effective training you perform
- How well you progress your exercises over time

Some women improve their pelvic floor muscle control within a couple of weeks of starting their exercises and so start to notice improved prolapse symptoms. Rapid gains in strength can often be made at the outset of pelvic floor training programs. If your pelvic floor is deconditioned you will need to be prepared to put time and effort into your training. Pelvic floor exercises should be performed regularly for at least 5 months to achieve strength changes and functional improvements.[7] Commitment to regular pelvic floor exercises will help you to maintain your pelvic floor support and prevent pelvic floor deconditioning that occurs without regular pelvic floor exercise and increasing age.

How to Get 'The Knack'

'The Knack' is an exercise technique that can support and protect your pelvic floor. It involves contracting your pelvic floor muscles before and during episodes of increased pelvic floor loading. When performed correctly, 'The Knack' may help you to reduce pelvic floor stretch and strain during large increases in pressure on your pelvic floor. In doing so it may help to prevent worsening of your prolapse or reduce the risk of repeat prolapse after prolapse surgery.

To perform 'The Knack' lift and squeeze your pelvic floor muscles before and during intense pelvic floor loading that occurs with cough, sneeze or heavy lifting. To be effective, this technique needs to be well timed to start before any downward pressure on your pelvic floor - it's too late to start contracting your pelvic floor muscles during the loading event.

Pelvic Floor Training and Prolapse Surgery

Pelvic floor exercises are often recommended for women before and after prolapse surgery. Pelvic floor training aims to improve pelvic floor support for surgery and minimise the risk of repeat prolapse. Some women develop pelvic floor problems such as bladder leakage as a result of prolapse surgery and pelvic floor exercise aims to minimise the risk of these types of post-operative problems.

Pelvic floor training before prolapse surgery

It seems reasonable to assume that learning the correct pelvic floor exercise technique and 'The Knack' before prolapse surgery should improve your ability to exercise and protect your pelvic floor post-operatively. Pre-operative pelvic floor muscle strengthening may promote improved pelvic floor support following surgery, however this remains to be confirmed by scientific studies.

Pre-operative pelvic floor physiotherapy can help you prepare for prolapse surgery. During your consultation you can usually expect to learn the correct pelvic floor exercise technique and guidelines for pre-operative pelvic floor training. Your exercise program will be tailored to your current level of ability - there is no one pelvic floor exercise program for every woman. Pre-operative pelvic floor exercise is usually prescribed along the lines of the daily pelvic floor exercise routine outlined earlier in this chapter. Your physiotherapist may also help you identify and better manage potential post-operative risks such as poor bowel habits.

Pelvic floor exercises after prolapse surgery

Your post-operative pelvic floor exercises will be directed by your surgeon. When to commence exercises will be determined according to the type of prolapse surgery performed, your rate of recovery and any post-operative complications you may experience. This may be around 4-6 weeks after surgery, but varies, so be guided by your surgeon's instructions. If you are unsure about when to commence your exercises ask your physiotherapist or nursing staff for your surgeon's guidelines prior to your discharge from hospital.

Tips for pelvic floor exercises after prolapse surgery:

- Pelvic floor exercises should always be pain free - if you experience pelvic floor discomfort during or after your exercises, you may be using the wrong technique, or overdoing things, so stop, rest and recover. If discomfort with pelvic floor exercise persists, cease your exercises and speak with your doctor or physiotherapist before proceeding.
- Focus on using the correct pelvic floor exercise technique when you first commence pelvic floor exercises after surgery. It's important to avoid downward pressure on your pelvic floor with the wrong exercise technique. Knowing how to

perform your pelvic floor exercises prior to surgery can help ensure correct post-operative technique.

- Relax your pelvic floor muscles completely back to their normal resting length after every exercise. Some women tend to habitually overbrace their pelvic floor muscles. Over bracing can sometimes occur as a result of pelvic discomfort after pelvic floor surgery in which case the initial focus should be learning to relax the pelvic floor muscles before strengthening.
- Perform your pelvic floor exercises when your body is rested rather than fatigued. A comfortable position for resting and reducing pelvic floor pressure is lying down with a pillow beneath the knees.
- Choose antigravity positions for your exercises when starting out. Lying down on your back with a pillow beneath your knees or side lying with a pillow between your legs, are suitable antigravity positions that can help you gradually recommence your pelvic floor exercises.
- Progress your pelvic floor exercises gradually over time. It will usually take some time before you are able to do your exercises at your pre-operative intensity. Listen to your body and gradually increase the strength of your contractions, the number of repetitions and the length of your exercises as your pelvic floor recovers.
- Use 'The Knack' to protect your prolapse during episodes of pelvic floor loading after your prolapse repair.

Key Points for Prolapse Support Exercises

- ♀ Pelvic floor exercises can reduce prolapse symptoms and severity in some women.
- ♀ The risk of repeat prolapse is increased following prolapse surgery.
- ♀ Your pelvic floor muscles sit in layers, in and around the area where you sit.
- ♀ Pelvic floor muscles play an important role in supporting pelvic organs against prolapse.
- ♀ It is important to understand the correct pelvic floor exercise technique from the outset of training.
- ♀ Correct pelvic floor exercise technique involves an inwards lift and squeeze, in and around all three pelvic openings, followed by relaxation of the pelvic floor muscles back to normal resting levels.
- ♀ To strengthen your pelvic floor aim for 3 sets of 8-12 strong pelvic floor exercises, maintaining each exercise up to 10 seconds, followed by 10 brisk pelvic floor exercises every day.
- ♀ Progress your pelvic floor exercises over time for ongoing pelvic floor strengthening.
- ♀ The intensity of effort or strength of pelvic floor muscle contractions is important for pelvic floor strengthening.
- ♀ It can take 5 months of regular pelvic floor exercise to reveal an effect.

- ♀ 'The Knack' is a protective pre-contraction of the pelvic floor muscles before and during increased downward pressure upon the pelvic floor.
- ♀ Pelvic floor training before surgery is desirable to learn correct pelvic floor exercise technique, optimise pelvic floor condition and learn 'The Knack'.
- ♀ Post-operative pelvic floor exercises should be commenced and progressed according to your surgeon's guidelines.
- ♀ Pelvic floor exercises after prolapse surgery should be pain free and gradually progressed.
- ♀ Commitment to regular pelvic floor exercises after prolapse surgery will help to maintain long-term pelvic floor muscle support.
- ♀ If you are unsure about pelvic floor exercises with a prolapse or after prolapse surgery seek professional guidance from a trained pelvic floor physiotherapist.

Section II

Strength & Fitness Exercises

3 Exercising for Your Weakest Link

Everybody is different and no one exercise program can perfectly suit every woman. Women with well functioning pelvic floor support may be able perform most regular physical fitness exercises without pelvic floor problems. Other women who are at increased risk of pelvic floor dysfunction are better suited to pelvic floor safe exercises that reduce their risk of worsening pelvic floor problems with exercise. Some physical activities and exercises will be appropriate for some women and inappropriate for others.

General Exercise for Prolapse

Ideally your exercises should be appropriate for your weakest link. For many women with pelvic organ prolapse, the weakest physical link is their pelvic floor, or more specifically the supportive capacity of their pelvic floor. If you have a prolapse, you are likely to have pelvic floor weakness or dysfunction. This means your pelvic floor is more vulnerable to injury than that of a woman with well functioning pelvic floor support.

If you have a pelvic prolapse, or previous prolapse surgery, your general exercises should be appropriate for how well your pelvic floor is currently supporting your pelvic organs. Matching your exercises to your current level of pelvic support ensures that your pelvic floor can withstand the increased loading that occurs with general exercise. This will help you exercise and minimise prolapse symptoms, reduce your risk of pelvic floor overload and help you protect your prolapse or prolapse repair.

Pelvic Floor Overload with Exercise

When you are upright the load on your pelvic floor increases - this is a normal, unavoidable part of everyday living. When you stand upright, the downward force of gravity combines with the weight of your abdomen to increase the load placed down onto your pelvic floor. Your pelvic floor muscles and internal supporting tissues work together to retain your pelvic organs in their correct position and withstand this load.

Unfortunately some general exercises and techniques can increase the load on the pelvic floor to the extent where they overload the pelvic floor - especially in women who are at increased risk of prolapse. If the downward forces associated with your exercises exceed the load your pelvic floor can withstand, then your pelvic floor will be forced downwards.

When the pelvic floor is repeatedly loaded over time, or with one particularly intense episode of loading such as lifting a very heavy weight, the pelvic floor can be overstretched and strained.

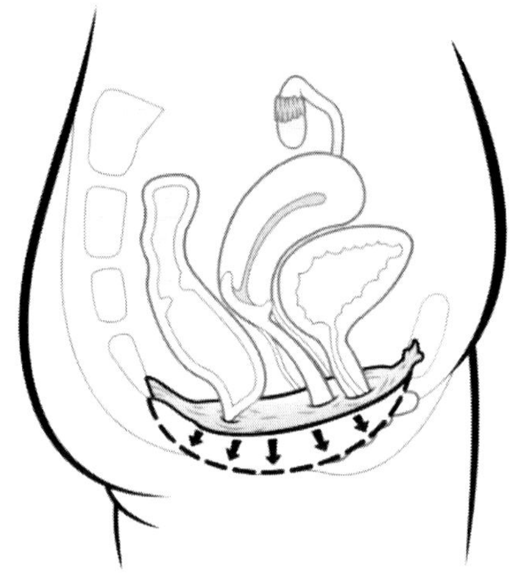

Pelvic Floor Descent

Overstretching causes the pelvic floor muscles and tissues become weak and less able to withstand the loading forces associated with exercise. This is how some exercises can overload the pelvic floor contributing to worsening prolapse symptoms or even repeat prolapse after prolapse surgery.

Knowing Your Individual Risks

If you have a prolapse, or have had prolapse surgery you are likely to have some weakness or deficit in your pelvic floor supporting structures. Exercises that place more stress on your pelvic floor than it can withstand can potentially worsen existing pelvic floor problems and increase your risk of prolapse.

Inappropriate exercises pose more risk to some women with prolapse than others, especially women with one or more risk factors for prolapse (outlined in Chapter 1). For example, if you have a prolapse, and you are overweight, your abdominal weight increases the load on your pelvic floor during upright exercises. If you've had prolapse surgery your risk of repeat pelvic floor prolapse is increased. Your exercise program should be modified according to your specific risks to allow you to exercise and avoid undue strain on your pelvic floor.

How Much to Modify Your Exercises

Understanding how well your pelvic floor is supporting your internal organs can help you know how much you need to modify your exercise program. A woman with a mild prolapse and strong, well functioning pelvic floor muscles may be able to perform a wider range of more intense physical exercises than a woman with a moderate prolapse and poorly functioning pelvic floor support. If you're not sure how well your pelvic floor muscles are working for support, seek a consultation with a pelvic floor physiotherapist who can provide you with this information.

Some women don't have access to pelvic floor physiotherapy. If you are in this situation, knowing how much you need to modify exercises can be challenging. As a general guide, if you have a pelvic prolapse, or if you are at increased risk of prolapse then err on the side of caution and avoid or modify those exercises and techniques known to substantially increase pelvic floor loading. A range of pelvic floor safe exercises and techniques, along with exercises requiring caution, are outlined in the following chapters.

General Guide to Exercise with Prolapse Problems

The following key points are expanded upon throughout this book.

Pelvic floor support
Improve and maintain your pelvic floor muscle support with regular pelvic floor exercise. If your pelvic floor muscles are weak and not functioning well, improving the condition of your pelvic floor with regular pelvic floor or Kegel exercises is essential. As your overall pelvic floor condition improves, so too can your capacity to do a wider range of exercises and intensities.

Manage your risks
Know your individual risks for prolapse and manage those risk factors that you can control. If your individual risks place you at increased likelihood of pelvic floor strain or repeat prolapse then modify your exercise program to reduce potential strain accordingly.

Exercise for your weakest link
If your pelvic floor is your weakest link, then choose those exercises best suited to the strength and capacity of your pelvic floor and modify or avoid those exercises more likely to cause overload and injury.

Pelvic floor safe exercises
Pelvic floor safe exercises are those exercises and techniques that promote the individual ability of a woman to exercise and minimise the risk of pelvic floor overload. Adopting these exercises and techniques as part of your long-term prolapse management strategy can help you continue to exercise, decrease exercise-related prolapse symptoms and reduce the load on your pelvic floor.

Listen to your symptoms
Your prolapse symptoms can be a good indicator of those exercises or techniques that may be overloading your pelvic floor. Notice your prolapse symptoms during and after exercise and modify or avoid exercises that increase your symptoms. If you've had prolapse surgery try to recall those exercises that previously exacerbated your

prolapse symptoms - these are likely to be exercises with techniques to modify or avoid in the future.

Medical guidance
Seek guidance from your treating doctor or pelvic floor health professional if you have a prolapse and feel uncertain about general exercise. It's important to follow medical guidelines regarding your exercises and to adhere to post-operative prolapse surgery exercise instructions.

When to See Your Doctor Prior to Exercise?

Exercising safely involves knowing when to seek a medical review before starting a new exercise program. This following information is designed to give you insight into your own readiness for exercise and whether or not you require pre-exercise medical assessment. If you are unsure about your individual capacity for exercise, seek an assessment with your doctor prior to commencing any new exercise program.

Women with prolapse problems
If you have a prolapse, consultation with a pelvic floor physiotherapist prior to commencing a new exercise program can help you understand your individual risks and the capacity of your pelvic floor to cope with general exercise. If you've had prolapse surgery seek your surgeon's approval before starting or recommencing general exercise. If you've had a recent prolapse repair it is particularly important that your body has sufficiently healed before recommencing general exercises.

Pre-exercise screening
If you are over the age of 65 years old, or if you have a chronic health condition that requires regular medical treatment, seek your doctor's approval to exercise and develop a physical activity plan with a health professional. Women over 55 years of age are generally considered to be at higher risk of heart disease and may need to see a doctor prior to exercise.

Key Points for General Exercise and Prolapse

- ♀ The pelvic floor is often the weakest link for women with prolapse.
- ♀ If your pelvic floor is your weakest link then adopt a pelvic floor safe exercise program.
- ♀ Some women are at greater risk of prolapse problems with exercise than others.
- ♀ Women who have had prolapse surgery are at increased risk of repeat prolapse and should adopt pelvic floor safe exercises long-term.
- ♀ Know your individual risk factors for prolapse and exercise, so you can modify your general exercises according to your level of risk.
- ♀ Pelvic floor overload is a risk for women seeking to exercise with a prolapse or after prolapse surgery.
- ♀ Pelvic floor overload can cause pelvic floor weakness and worsen prolapse problems.
- ♀ Improve your pelvic floor support with regular pelvic floor exercises to promote your ability to stay active with a prolapse.
- ♀ Listen to your body and avoid or modify exercises that exacerbate your prolapse symptoms.
- ♀ Be guided by your treating doctor or pelvic floor health professional about the capacity of your pelvic floor for general exercises.
- ♀ Seek your surgeon's approval before starting or recommencing general exercise if you've had prolapse surgery.
- ♀ If you are over the age of 65 years old, or if you have a chronic health condition that requires regular medical treatment, seek your doctor's approval to exercise and develop a physical activity plan with a health professional.

4 Strength Exercises and Prolapse

Strength training is also known as resistance training. Strength training typically involves contracting muscles repeatedly against some form of resistance, usually for the purpose of increasing physical strength. Resistance for strength exercises may be provided by free weights (e.g. dumbbells), weight machines, resistance bands, body weight or water (aquatic exercise).

Pelvic Floor Safe Strength Training

Pelvic floor safe strength training can help you strengthen your body and protect your pelvic floor. There is no one-fits-all rule when it comes to strength training with a prolapse. If you have prolapse problems, your individual capacity to perform pelvic floor safe strength training exercises is determined by your:

- Pelvic floor support
- Prolapse severity
- History of prolapse repair surgery
- General physical strength
- Experience with resistance training exercises

Many women with prolapse and those with well functioning pelvic floor muscles after prolapse repair, are capable of performing pelvic floor safe strength training exercises. Strength training may not be an appropriate form of exercise for some women with poor pelvic floor support, severe prolapse or prolapse repair - alternative forms of exercise may be more suitable.

Benefits of Strength Training for Women

Strength training has numerous potential benefits for women, especially during menopause and beyond. Established benefits of strength training include:

- Increased physical strength and endurance
- Increased lean muscle and muscle tone
- Improved bone health and reduced fracture risk
- Chronic disease prevention or management (e.g. diabetes, cardiovascular disease, osteoarthritis)
- Improved ability to perform everyday tasks
- Reduced anxiety and fatigue
- Improved energy levels

Potential Risks Associated with Strength Training

As with many forms of exercise there are potential risks for the pelvic floor associated with strength training. The main risk with strength training exercise relates to pelvic floor overload. This means that some aspect of the strength exercise creates too much pressure for the pelvic floor to withstand. When the pelvic floor is overloaded it is forced downwards, causing the pelvic floor tissues to stretch and weaken, potentially worsening prolapse problems.

Pelvic floor overload with strength training may be more likely with:

- Heavy loading or resistance
- Breath holding and straining
- Inappropriate strength exercises
- Inappropriate strength training techniques
- Inappropriate strength training positions

Pelvic floor safe strength training aims to help women perform strength exercises and avoid or reduce the risk of pelvic floor overload.

10 Step Guide to Pelvic Floor Safe Strength Training for Prolapse

This guide to pelvic floor safe strength training outlines the main principles for pelvic floor protection with strength exercise. This guide was first published in Inside Out[9] and the principles are adapted here for women with prolapse.

1. *Avoid heavy lifting*

Keep your weights or resistance levels within a manageable range. Any load that makes you strain or inclined to hold your breath is too heavy and should be decreased. If you've had prolapse surgery never lift more than the maximum lifting weight advised by your surgeon. Lifting weight from waist height or above is preferable to lifting weights from ground level - avoid lifting weights from the ground level wherever possible.

2. *Lift with good posture*

Maintain the normal inward curve in your lower back during the effort of your strength exercise i.e. lift, push or pull. The correct alignment of your spine will promote the protective activity of your supportive deep abdominal and pelvic floor muscles.

3. *Maximise pelvic floor support*

Activate your pelvic floor muscles before and during more intense resistance exercises. Some women with prolapse may choose to use a support pessary to help improve pelvic floor support. Adhere to your regular pelvic floor strength training exercises to maximise your pelvic floor capacity to withstand the pressure associated with your resistance exercises.

4. *Exhale with the effort*

Breathe out with the effort of your exercise, whether it is a lift, push or pull, to reduce the pressure on your pelvic floor. Avoid holding your breath as you use your muscles against a load. Breath holding and straining with resistance exercises will increase the downward pressure upon your pelvic floor.

5. *Choose supported positions*

Perform your resistance exercises sitting or lying down where possible, to eliminate the added force of gravity on your pelvic floor. Sitting on an exercise ball is an excellent option while you perform free weight or resistance band strength exercises.

6. *Avoid intense abdominal bracing*

Avoid strong abdominal bracing during resistance training exercises. Intense abdominal bracing will increase downward pressure on your pelvic floor. Correct abdominal bracing involves very gentle activation of the deep core abdominal muscles. Intense abdominal bracing will not improve prolapse support or flatten your lower abdomen.

7. *Progress gradually*

Focus your initial efforts on doing your exercises with the correct technique before adding resistance. Progress strength training exercises with the lightest available weight or resistance increments. Gradually increase resistance over time and only when you feel confident in your exercise technique and your improved pelvic floor muscle support.

8. *Take care when fatigued and rest*

When you are very tired, unwell or with lower back pain your pelvic floor muscles may not work as effectively for support and you may be more prone to prolapse symptoms or injury. Take a break and return to resistance training when you have recovered. Ensure adequate rest and recovery between resistance exercises. A time efficient way of allowing muscle recovery is to alternate your strength exercises - resting one muscle group while you exercise a different muscle group.

9. *Time your exercises*

Short regular bouts of resistance training are just as effective as longer sessions and may help you manage prolapse symptoms. If you are troubled by prolapse symptoms with exercise, or when returning to exercise after prolapse surgery you may find that a couple of short sessions spread out during the day, or over a couple of days may help you exercise with increased comfort.

10. *Avoid or modify aggravating exercises*

Listen to your body and notice any prolapse symptoms during and after strength exercises. If you develop prolapse symptoms or if your symptoms are worse with a specific exercise, then modify that exercise or leave it out of your program and perform another exercise to strengthen the same area.

Sample Pelvic Floor Safe Exercises - Whole Body Workout

Following is a sample whole body general strength training routine. Modify or avoid any of the following strength exercises that cause any prolapse symptoms or physical discomfort - remember every woman is different so that no one exercise program fits all. For demonstration and Physiotherapist guidance of these exercises refer to Pelvic Exercises Workout DVD.[8]

Mini Squat - hips, thighs and buttocks

- Stand with your feet approximately hip width apart
- Bend your knees and incline your trunk forwards
- Ensure that you can see your toes in front of your knees throughout
- Maintain the inward curve in your lower back
- Push down through your heels to return your trunk to upright
- Progress by holding dumbbell weights in front of your hips.

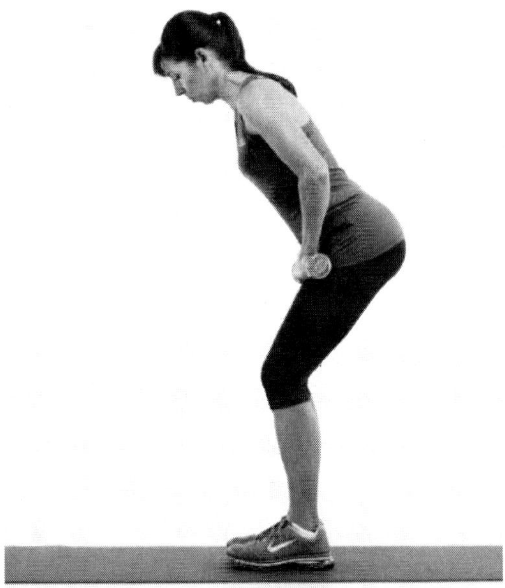

Pelvic floor safe tips:

- Avoid deep wide squats
- Breathe out as you return to standing upright
- Keep the dumbbell weight within a manageable range

Standing Forward Lunge - thighs and buttocks

- Stand with your feet astride in long lunge position
- Keep your trunk upright throughout
- Bend your knees lowering your back knee towards the ground
- Push down through the ball of your back foot to return to starting position
- Progress by holding dumbbell weights in front of your hips

Pelvic floor safe tips

- Avoid deep lunges
- Breathe out as you return to standing
- Keep the dumbbell weight within a manageable range

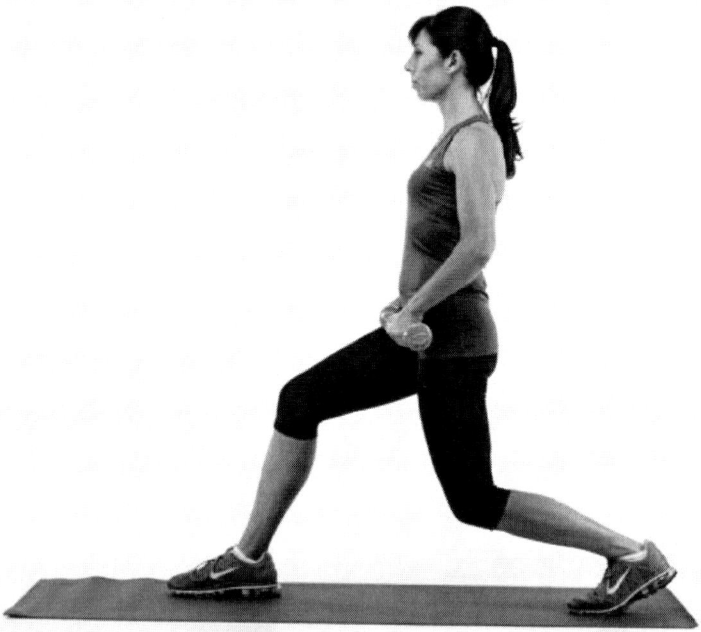

Calf Raise - calf muscles

- Stand tall feet slightly apart
- Hold onto the upright back of a chair or wall if unsteady
- Raise your heels off the ground to stand on the balls of your feet
- Lower your heels back to the ground
- Release your grip on the chair if you feel sufficiently confident in your balance to do calf raises without support
- Progress calf raises by holding dumbbell weights in front of your hips

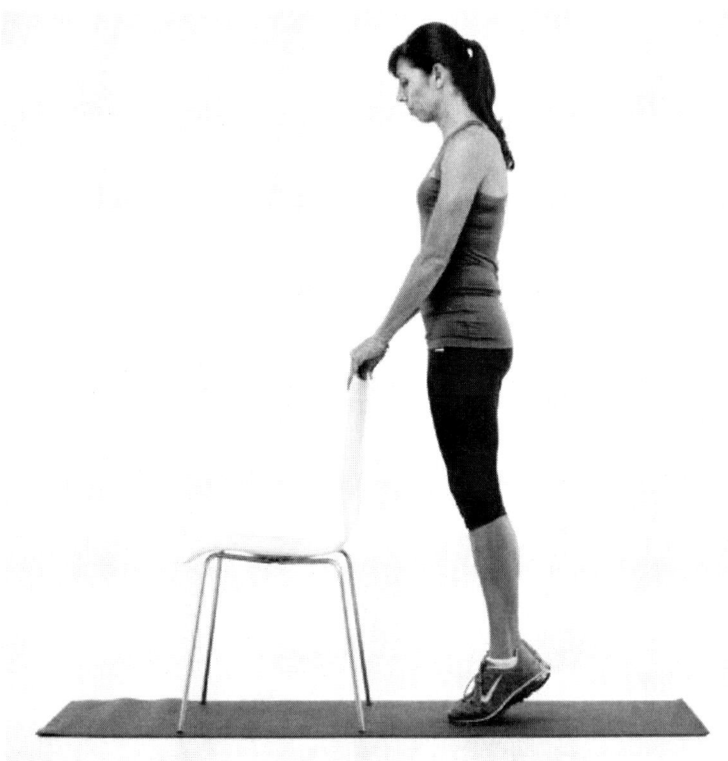

Low Dumbbell Row - middle back and shoulder

- Lean forward supporting your body with your left hand resting on a bench or exercise ball
- Hold your dumbbell weight in your right hand
- Raise the dumbbell along the outside line of your thigh
- Feel your right shoulder blade move inwards towards your spine as you lift the dumbbell, avoid using your upper shoulder/neck muscles and keep your gaze directed downwards
- Slowly lower the weight back to starting position

Pelvic floor safe tips

- Keep the dumbbell weight within a manageable range
- Breathe out as you lift the dumbbell

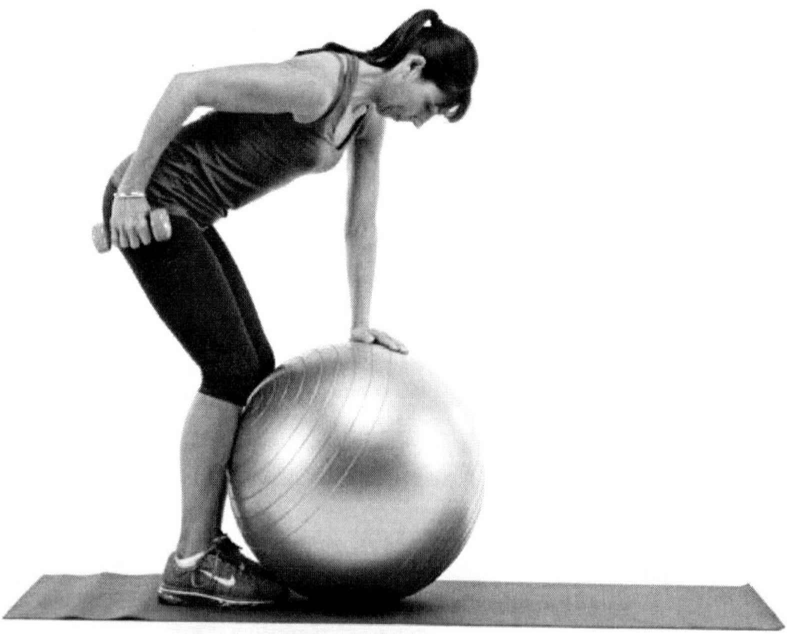

Seated Biceps Curl - front of upper arm

- Sit on a chair, stool or exercise ball
- Hold your dumbbell weights in both hands with your arms fully extended by your sides
- Sit tall lifting the crown of your head towards the ceiling
- Raise the dumbbell in your right hand towards your right shoulder
- Lower your right dumbbell back to your starting position
- Keep both elbows tucked into your waist throughout
- Repeat the same action lifting the left dumbbell towards your left shoulder
- Continue alternating arms

Pelvic floor safe tips:

- Raise one dumbbell at a time to minimise the load
- Breathe out when raising the dumbbell
- Keep the dumbbell weight within a manageable range

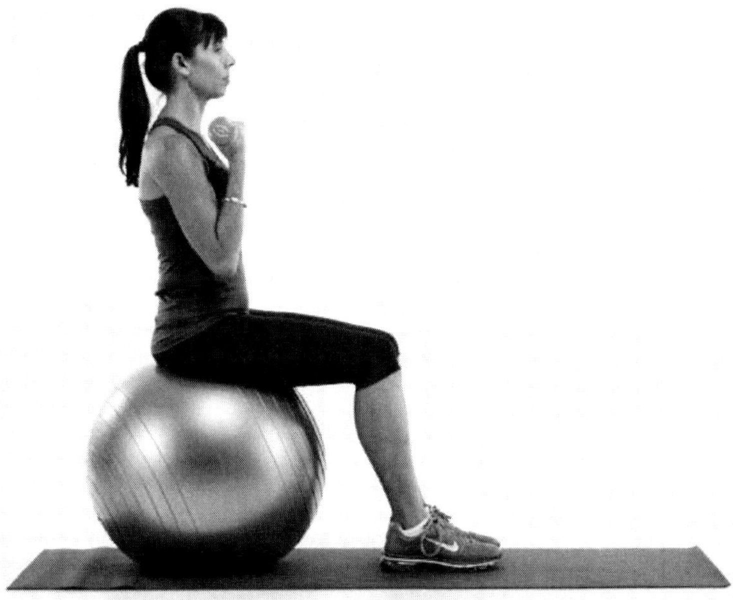

Triceps Extension - back of upper arm

- Sit on a chair, stool or exercise ball
- Hold your dumbbell weight in your right hand
- Lean forward resting your left forearm across your thighs to support your trunk
- Tuck your right upper arm into the right side of your body
- Hold your right elbow high throughout and keep your gaze directed downwards
- Extend your right arm by moving your dumbbell backwards
- Lower your dumbbell back to starting position
- Focus on using the muscles in the back of your upper arm rather than your neck and upper shoulder muscles

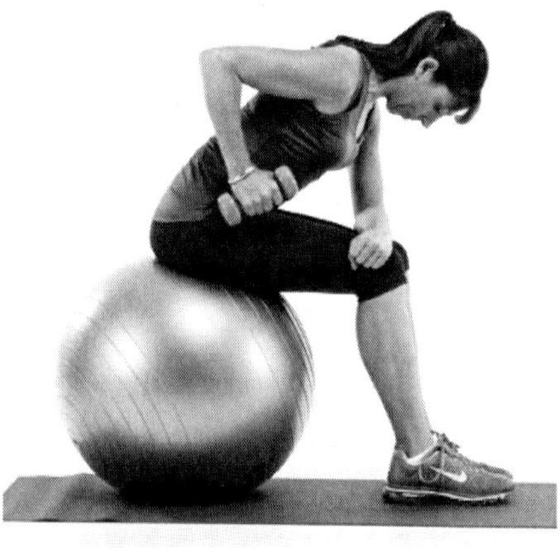

Triceps extension - start position

Triceps extension - elbow extended

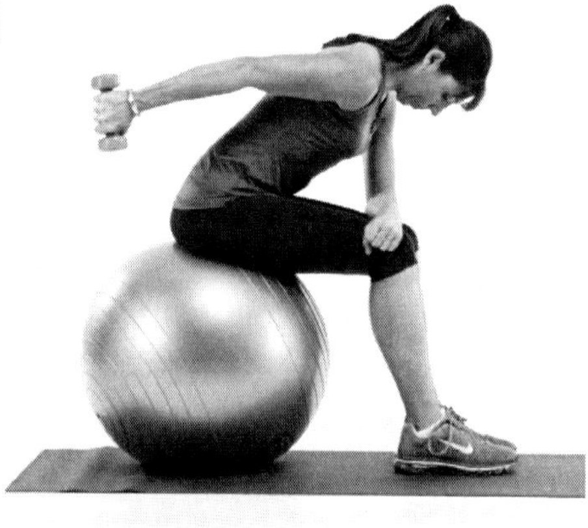

Pelvic floor safe tips:

- Keep the dumbbell weight within a manageable range

Floor Bridge - buttocks and lower back

- Lie down on your back on a firm surface
- Position your heels close your buttocks
- Keep your heels down and feet flat
- Push down through your heels and raise your buttocks off the ground
- Lower your body back down to starting position
- Maintain the normal inward curve in your lower back throughout
- Progress by resting dumbbell weights on your hips

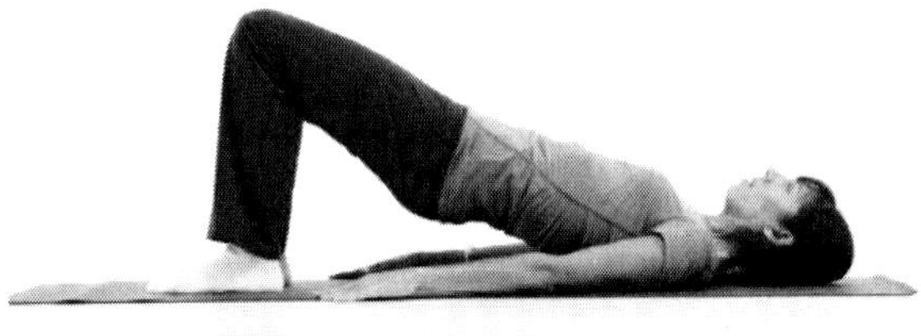

Pelvic floor safe tips:

- Breathe out when raising your body
- Keep the weight of your dumbbells within a manageable range

Alternate Arm Leg Raise - buttocks and lower back

- Lie down prone with a small cushion supporting your hips and pelvis
- Extend your left arm to reach in front of your body
- Raise your left arm and right leg together to just above ground level
- Slowly lower your limbs to starting position
- Repeat with your right arm and left leg
- Progress by keeping your limbs elevated above ground level for up to 30 second holds

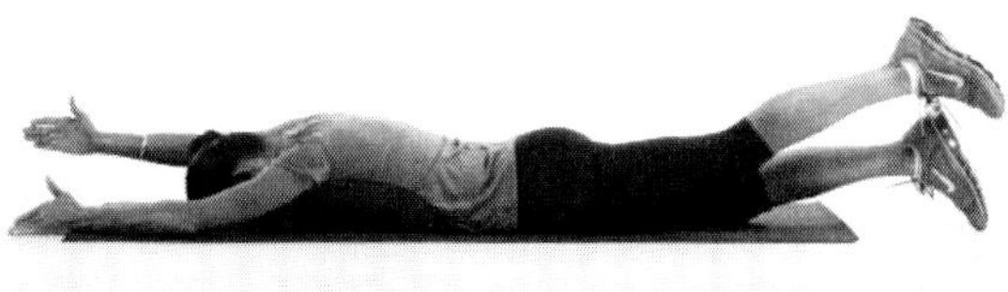

Strength Exercises Requiring Caution with Prolapse

Some strength exercises are more likely to increase pelvic floor loading and may need to be modified or avoided by some women with prolapse-related problems.

Strength exercises requiring caution include:

- Deep wide squats
- Deep forward or sideways lunges
- Dead lift with barbell
- Weighted leg press machine
- Standing squat machine
- Tricep dips
- Full men's push up
- High or weighted step down exercises
- Exercises supporting or lifting most of the body weight through the upper limbs
- Intense core abdominal exercises outlined in Chapter 6

Prolapse and Progressing Strength Exercises

Women with prolapse often feel limited when it comes to safely progressing strength exercises. Mainstream strength exercise programs usually rely upon progressively increasing the load (or resistance) to progress strengthening. Large increases in resistance are not the best option for women with prolapse, since heavy lifting is a known risk factor for prolapse.

There are alternatives to increasing the load to progress strength exercises. The effectiveness of a strength training program ultimately depends on the amount of strength exercise performed. The amount of strength exercise you perform is determined by a combination of factors i.e. how often you exercise, quantity (how many exercises), intensity (resistance or load), and resting time. To progress your strength exercises you may choose to:

- Increase the number of individual exercises or repetitions you perform up to 10-20 repetitions per set

- Gradually decrease the time spent resting between sets of exercise
- Perform single arm upper body exercises to allow for increased loading e.g. single arm biceps curls as opposed to double arm curls
- Gradually increase resistance with smallest possible increments in weight or resistance

General Muscle Strength Guidelines for Healthy Adults

The following strength training guidelines for healthy adults are provided by the American College of Sports Medicine:[10]

Appropriate strength exercises

- Choose a variety of strength exercises using a range of equipment including dumbbell weights, resistance bands or exercise machines
- Include exercises for the major muscle groups.

Frequency

- 2-3 times per week allowing muscle groups to rest for 48-72 hours between resistance training sessions.

Quantity

- 8-12 repeated exercises (repetitions) of each exercise
- 2-4 groups (sets) of repeated exercises for each muscle group
- Rest for 2-3 minutes between each set to allow muscle recovery.

Intensity

- Strength exercises should induce muscle fatigue rather than exhaustion
- Very light to light intensity is more appropriate for older adults or individuals who are deconditioned (e.g. after illness)
- For individuals using lighter weights the number of repetitions can be gradually increased to 10-20 repeated exercises for each exercise
- Progressively increase resistance over time for ongoing strengthening.

Key Points for Strength Exercises and Prolapse

- ♀ Your individual capacity to perform strength exercises is determined by a number of factors including the level of support provided by your pelvic floor muscles.
- ♀ Strength training can provide women with numerous physical and emotional benefits.
- ♀ The risk of pelvic floor overload with strength training can be minimised with pelvic floor safe strength training principles.
- ♀ Adhere to the 10 step guide to pelvic floor safe strength training to minimise the risk of pelvic floor overload.
- ♀ There is no one-fits-all pelvic floor safe strength training program for women.
- ♀ Avoid or modify those strength exercises requiring caution including those exercises that contribute to your prolapse symptoms.
- ♀ To strengthen your muscles aim to perform 2-4 sets of 8-12 repeated exercises for the major muscle groups on 2-3 alternate week days.
- ♀ The intensity of resistance exercises or the load being lifted often needs to be modified by women with prolapse and alternative methods of progression used.
- ♀ Seek the approval of your surgeon before commencing strength training exercises after prolapse surgery.

5 Pelvic Floor Safe Abdominal Core Exercises for Prolapse

Your deepest innermost abdominal muscles wrap like a corset around your trunk - these muscles should ideally work with your pelvic floor muscles. They are called the Transverse Abdominis muscles. When these muscles contract in coordination with other muscles surrounding your trunk including your pelvic floor muscles, they help to control the pressure within your abdomen. These lower deep abdominal muscles are the most appropriate abdominal muscles to exercise if you have a prolapse.

How to Exercise Deep Abdominal Core Muscles

There are some important steps to work through when correctly exercising your deep core abdominal muscles:

1. Setting your posture
2. Finding your deep abdominal muscles
3. Activating your deep abdominal muscles
4. Training your deep abdominal muscles

Correct Posture for Deep Abdominal Exercises

The first step in exercising your lower deep abdominal muscles is to position your spine into the correct posture, particularly the alignment of your lower back. The position in which your deep abdominal muscles will work most effectively is known as neutral spine position.

Neutral spine position lying down:

- Lie down on your back with your knees bent and feet flat
- Lengthen your spine
- Look straight at the ceiling so that your eyes and nose face forward
- Tuck your chin slightly
- Bring your shoulder blades back towards your spine and slightly down, so that your upper spine is quite straight
- Position your lower back so that it has a slight inward curve, or a space between the supporting surface and your lower back (shown over). Neutral is the midway position between arching your lower back and flattening it out completely

Neutral spine posture in upright positions (sitting or standing) is found using these same basic guidelines for positioning your spine. This is the best posture for exercising your deep abdominal muscles when you are sitting or standing.

How to Find your Deep Abdominal Muscles

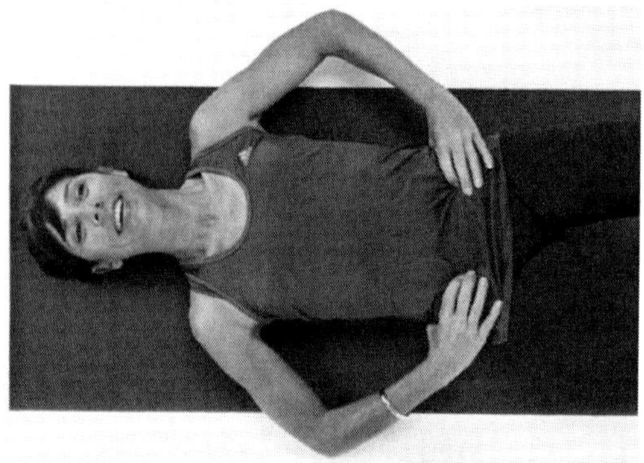

Finding your deep abdominal muscles can be challenging when you first start out. Your deepest abdominal muscles are positioned beneath layers of abdominal muscles and other tissues.

When you activate your deep lower abdominal muscles focus your attention on your lower abdominal wall, beneath the area where a pair of full briefs would sit over your lower abdomen. The best position to feel your deep abdominal muscles with your fingers is just inside your pelvic bones. If you wrap your thumbs and forefingers around your waist, your fingers will rest directly above your deep abdominal muscles, just inside your pelvic bones.

How to Activate your Deep Abdominal Muscles

Correct technique for deep abdominal muscle action involves gentle activation, however many women tend to overbrace these muscles at first. Try to avoid overbracing which can increase pressure on your pelvic floor.

To correctly activate your deep abdominal muscles:

- Lie down on your back with your spine in neutral position
- Slowly and gently draw your lower abdominal wall slightly inwards away from your briefs and towards your spine - this is a subtle movement rather than a strong contraction
- Keep your breathing regular as you contract your abdominal muscles for up to 10 seconds at a time or even longer with improved core abdominal muscle control
- You may be able to feel a subtle contraction of your abdominal wall beneath your forefingers with correct abdominal muscle activation. Your upper abdominal 'six-pack' muscles shouldn't contract strongly as you activate your lower deep abdominal muscles

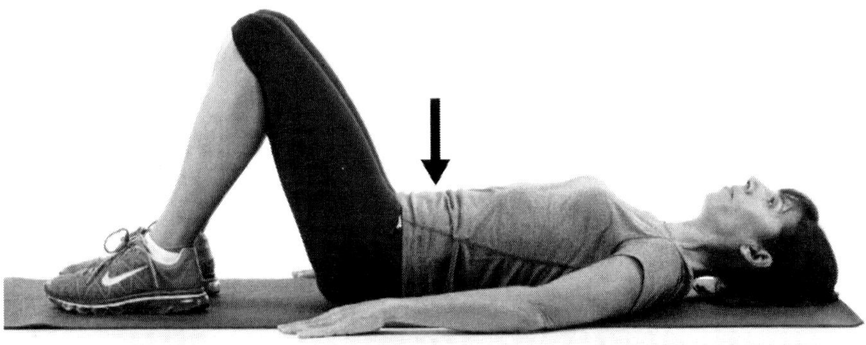

Neutral spine position -
arrow indicating direction of abdominal activation

Mistakes to Avoid with Deep Abdominal Exercises

Try to avoid these common mistakes during deep abdominal exercises:

- Slumped forwards posture
- Holding your breath
- Overbracing your abdominal muscles

Pelvic Floor Safe Abdominal Muscle Exercises

When you understand how to correctly activate your deep abdominal muscles, you are ready to progress to pelvic floor safe deep abdominal exercises. The following sample deep abdominal exercises include lying down and seated exercises with progressions to help you improve the condition of your deep abdominal muscles.

Lying Down Mat Abdominal Muscle Exercises

The following exercises are slow controlled, deep abdominal core muscle exercises. They are not always as easy as they look when performed correctly.

Heel Slides

- Start lying down on your back, knees bent and feet flat
- Use a cushion to support your head and neck as required
- Position your spine in neutral position
- Gently activate your deep abdominal muscles and maintain this contraction throughout this exercise
- Straighten one leg by slowly sliding your heel along the ground away from your buttocks
- Keep your spine and pelvis stable throughout - as soon as your lower back starts to arch upwards return your heel back to starting position
- Relax your abdominal muscles, rest briefly and repeat up to 10 heel slides for each leg

As your abdominal muscle control improves you may be able to slide your heel further away from your buttocks before your lower back starts to move.

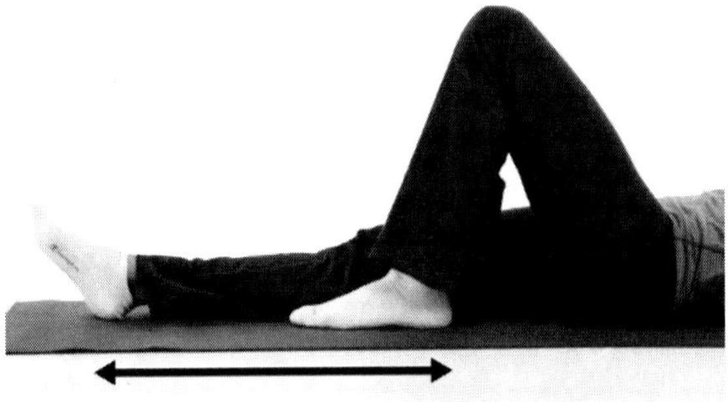

Bent Knee Fall Outs

- Start lying down on your back, knees bent and feet flat
- Use a cushion to support your neck as required
- Position your spine in neutral position
- Gently activate your lower abdominal muscles and maintain this contraction throughout
- Slowly lower one bent knee out to the side of your body away from your midline
- Keep your spine and pelvis stable throughout - as soon as you notice your trunk start to roll return your knee back towards your starting position

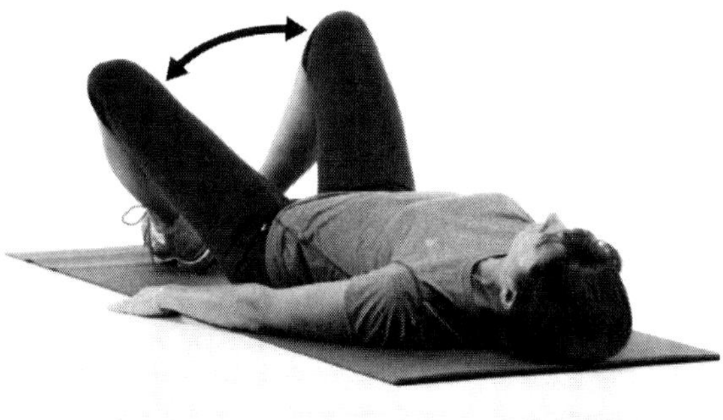

- Relax your abdominal muscles, rest briefly and repeat up to 10 bent knee fall outs for each leg

As your abdominal muscle control improves you will be able to lower your knee further away from your midline before your trunk starts to roll.

Single Leg Raises

- Single leg raises provide a pelvic floor safe alternative to double leg raise deep core abdominal exercises
- Start lying down on your back, knees bent and feet flat
- Use a cushion to support your neck, as required
- Position your spine in neutral position
- Gently activate your lower abdominal muscles and maintain this contraction throughout
- Slowly raise one bent leg towards the ceiling
- Keep your spine and pelvis stable throughout - as soon as your lower back starts to flatten out, or you feel your pelvis start to move, lower your foot back to your starting position
- Relax your abdominal muscles, rest briefly and repeat up to 10 single leg raises for each leg

As your abdominal control improves you will find you can raise your knee progressively higher before your lower back starts to flatten out.

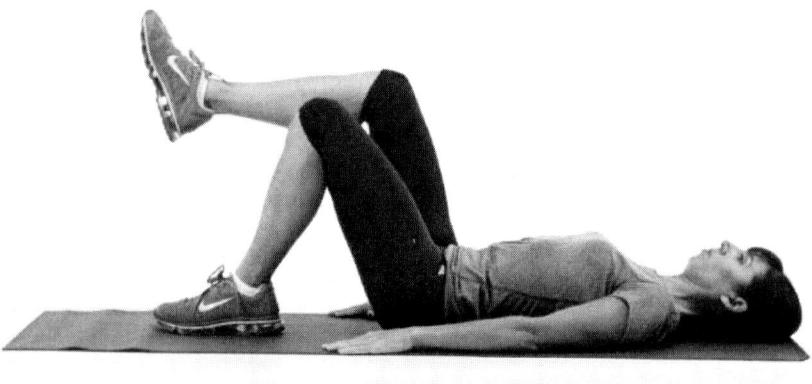

Seated Deep Abdominal Exercises

Seated exercises are an ideal way of training your deep abdominal core muscles to work when you are upright. These seated exercises can be performed sitting on a chair or on an exercise ball. The instability of an exercise ball creates additional challenge when performing and progressing these exercises.

Basic Seated Abdominal Muscle Exercise

This basic seated deep abdominal muscle exercise can be practiced sitting on a chair or an exercise ball. This exercise provides the basic technique from which the following seated abdominal exercises are progressed.

- Sit with your feet flat and your knees approximately hip width apart
- Your body weight should be evenly distributed between your sit bones
- Position your spine in neutral with the normal inward curve in your lower back
- Lift your chest and keep your spine tall
- Keep your eyes and nose facing forwards and your chin slightly tucked
- Slowly and gently activate your deep abdominal muscles using the technique already outlined (image over page)
- If unsure about your abdominal contraction, place your fingers just beside your pelvic bones to feel your lower abdominal wall tension slightly as you contract your deep abdominal muscles
- Breathe as you maintain your deep abdominal muscle contraction for up to 10 seconds
- Relax your abdominal muscles, rest briefly and repeat this exercise up to 10 times in a row

Progress your seated deep abdominal muscle exercises with the following deep abdominal exercises when you feel confident in your correct technique.

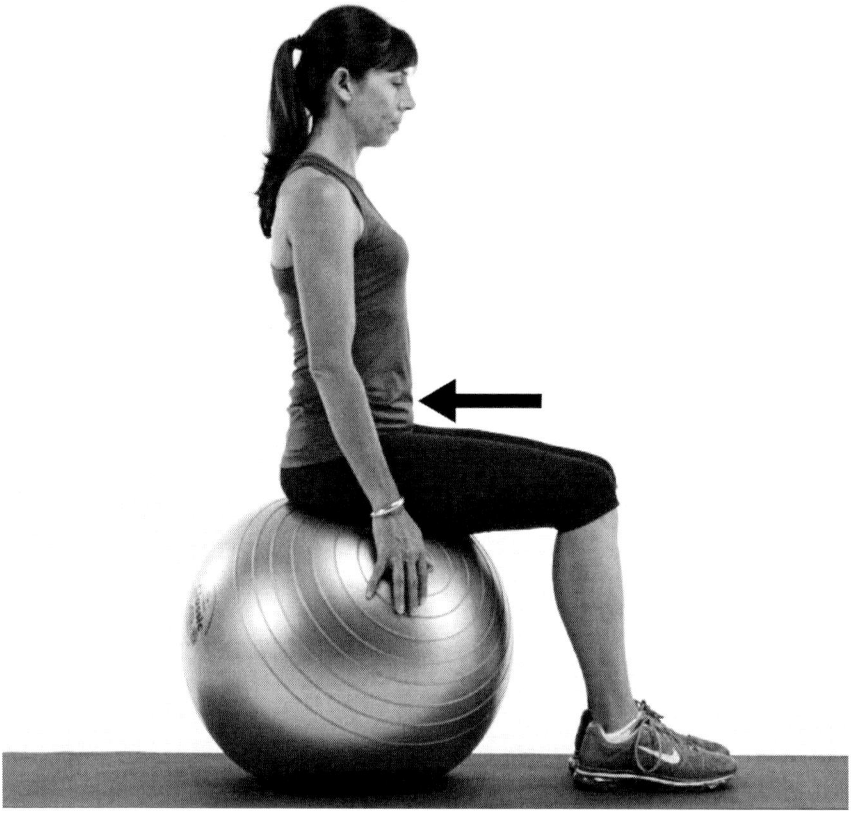

Basic seated abdominal exercise

Heel Digs

Heel digs are a progression exercise from the basic seated abdominal exercise.

- Sit and activate your deep abdominal muscles using the seated abdominal activation exercise guidelines
- Position your arms by your sides and if using an exercise ball hold onto the sides of the ball
- Slowly extend one leg to touch your heel to the ground in front of your body before returning your leg back to your starting position
- Maintain your deep abdominal muscle contraction throughout, keeping your weight evenly balanced through your sit bones and your pelvis stable
- Relax your abdominal muscles, rest briefly and repeat up to 10 heel digs for each leg

As your deep abdominal muscle control improves you can progress this exercise by decreasing your hand contact with the ball to holding with 1-2 fingers and then letting go of the ball altogether when you feel sufficiently stable and confident. The following exercises can all be progressed in this same manner.

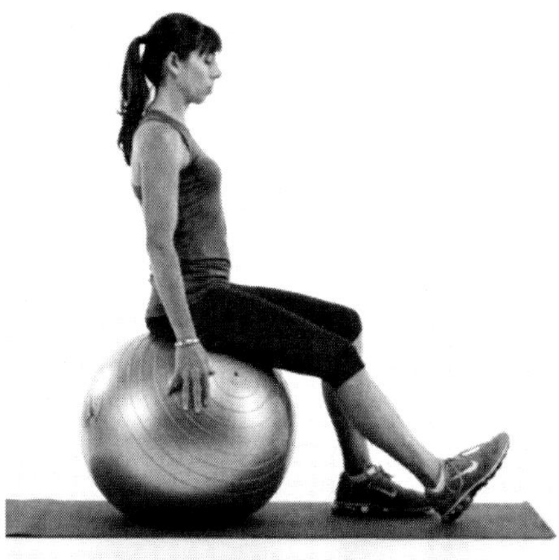

Knee Lifts

Knee lifts are a core abdominal exercise progression from heel digs.

- Sit and activate your deep abdominal muscles using the basic seated abdominal activation exercise guidelines
- Position your arms by your sides and if using an exercise ball hold onto the sides of the ball with all fingers
- Slowly raise one knee to lift one foot just off the ground in front of your body
- Lower your leg back to your starting position
- Maintain your deep abdominal muscle contraction throughout, keeping your weight evenly balanced through your sit bones and your pelvis stable
- Relax your abdominal muscles, rest briefly and repeat up to 10 knee lifts for each leg

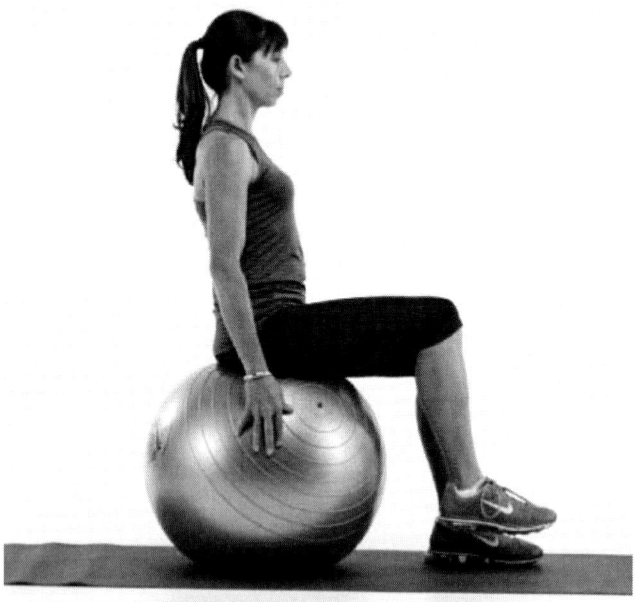

Knee Lift Leg Extend

This exercise provides a progression from seated knee lifts.

- Position your body as for knee lifts and activate your deep abdominal muscles using the basic seated abdominal control exercise guidelines
- Place your arms by your sides and if you are using an exercise ball hold onto the sides of the ball
- Raise one foot just off the ground in front of your body
- Keep your foot raised off the ground and extend your leg in front of your body
- Bend your knee before lowering your foot back to the ground
- Maintain your deep abdominal muscle contraction throughout, and keep your weight evenly balanced and your pelvis stable
- Relax your abdominal muscles, rest briefly and repeat up to 10 exercises for each leg

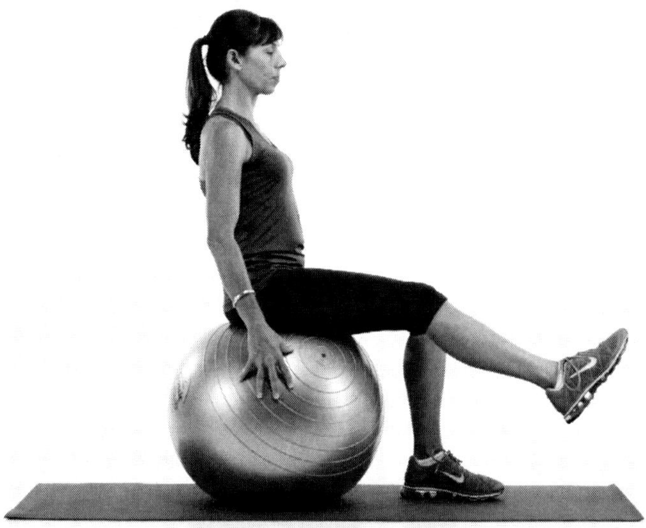

Key Points for Core Abdominal Exercises

- ♀ Pelvic floor safe deep abdominal muscle exercises are those exercises that train the abdominal core muscles and minimise pressure on the pelvic floor.
- ♀ Deep abdominal muscle exercises can improve the tone, support and control provided by the deepest corset-like abdominal muscles that wrap around the trunk.
- ♀ Your deep abdominal muscles should work in a balanced and coordinated manner with the muscles surrounding your trunk, including your pelvic floor.
- ♀ Effective deep abdominal muscle exercises require neutral spine posture.
- ♀ Correct activation of the deep abdominal muscles involves a gentle contraction of the muscles beneath the lower abdominal wall.
- ♀ Common mistakes to avoid with core abdominal exercises include overbracing the abdominal muscles, breath holding and slumped forwards posture.
- ♀ Deep abdominal muscle exercises are readily progressed for both lying down mat and seated upright exercises.

6 Abdominal Exercises and Pelvic Floor Overload

Knowing how to identify inappropriate abdominal exercises and choose pelvic floor safe alternatives is important if you are seeking to strengthen your abdominal muscles with a prolapse. Some commonly performed intense core strength abdominal exercises are inappropriate for some women with prolapse. This doesn't mean that if you have prolapse problems you need to cease all abdominal exercises. Rather, this means choosing the most appropriate core abdominal exercises and avoiding those abdominal exercises more likely to overload your pelvic floor.

Intense Abdominal Exercises and Pelvic Floor Muscles

Your pelvic floor muscles are designed to work with other muscles surrounding your trunk to manage the pressure within your abdomen. Ideally your pelvic floor and abdominal muscles should work together in a balanced and coordinated manner. Sometimes an imbalance develops between the pelvic floor and abdominal muscles and when this happens pelvic floor problems can develop or worsen.

There are two main pelvic floor problems that can arise from inappropriate abdominal exercises:

1. *Pelvic floor overload*

Women with prolapse often have pelvic floor muscle weakness and poor pelvic floor support. This means that their pelvic floor is unable to withstand strong downward pressure. Abdominal curl exercises are known to increase downward pressure on the pelvic floor. Studies show that when women with poorly functioning pelvic floor muscles perform abdominal curl exercises, their pelvic floor descends[11]. Repeated upper abdominal muscle exercises that continually force the pelvic floor downwards may cause progressive pelvic floor muscle stretch and weakness over time. With more intense upper abdominal strength exercises, there is more downward force upon the pelvic floor. This is one reason why prolapse symptoms can be associated with intense or repeated abdominal strength exercises.

2. *Pelvic floor overbracing*

If the pelvic floor muscles become overactive with too much core muscle contraction and insufficient relaxation, the risk of pelvic floor injury increases. It may seem a little contradictory, however if you have a prolapse and your pelvic floor muscles become too tight and unable to relax, your overall prolapse support will actually decrease.

Some women automatically contract their lower abdominal and pelvic floor muscles together during abdominal exercises. With sustained abdominal exercises, their pelvic floor muscles may become too tight and unable to relax. If the pelvic floor muscles become too tight, the pelvic floor becomes more susceptible to injury.

Are Intense Core Exercises Inappropriate for Everyone?

No, some women have strong, well functioning pelvic floor muscles that are capable of withstanding the pressure generated by intense core abdominal exercises. Pelvic floor exercise and rehabilitation may improve the capacity of your pelvic floor to cope with more advanced core abdominal exercises over time. If you've had prolapse surgery keep your core abdominal exercises within a manageable level of intensity and avoid overloading your pelvic floor.

If you have prolapse problems, the intensity of your core abdominal strength exercises should match your pelvic floor support.

How to Identify Intense Core Abdominal Exercises to Avoid?

Intense core abdominal strength exercises exist in many women's exercise programs. The core exercises most likely to overload the pelvic floor are intense upper abdominal muscle exercises because these muscles generate a lot of downward force.

The following intense core abdominal strength exercises are grouped into categories for ease of understanding. This list is by no means exhaustive and is intended as a general guide to help you understand how to identify and avoid intense core abdominal exercises.

Head and Trunk Forward Raises

Exercises lifting the head and upper torso directly forwards off the supporting surface:

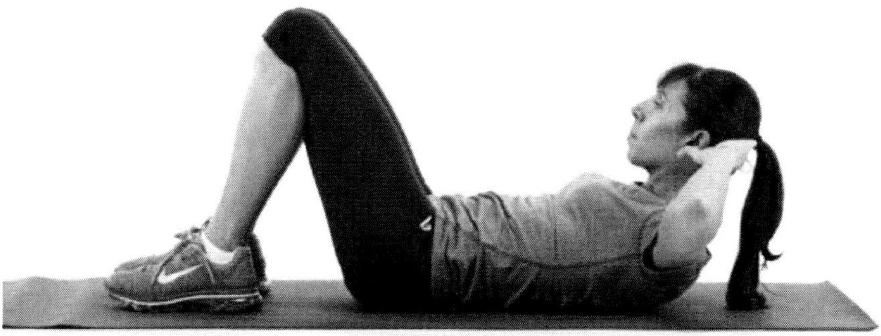

Abdominal curl

- Abdominal curl/crunch
- Long arm crunch
- Exercise ball/Swiss ball crunch
- Weighted crunch
- Incline sit ups
- Vertical leg crunch

Double Leg Raises

Exercises where both legs are raised simultaneously off the supporting surface:

- Reverse crunch
- Flutter kicks
- Bicycle legs
- Tabletop (Pilates)
- Exercise ball or Swiss ball raises with legs

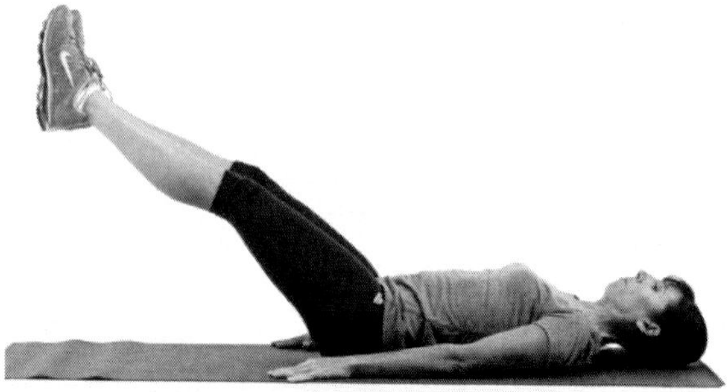

Upper Body and Double Leg Raises

Exercises where the legs, head and shoulders are raised simultaneously off the supporting surface:

- Vertical leg crunch
- V sits (Yoga)
- The Hundred (Pilates)

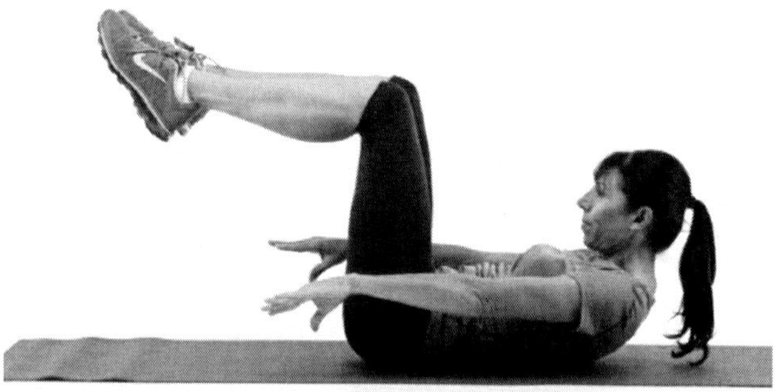

Weight Bearing Through the Upper Limbs

Exercises where the upper limbs support a large amount of body weight:

- Full men's push ups
- Tricep dips
- Chin ups
- Ball pikes
- Ball plank
- Roll out with forearms on ball
- Full plank (weight bearing through hands and feet)
- Full hover (weight bearing through forearms and feet)

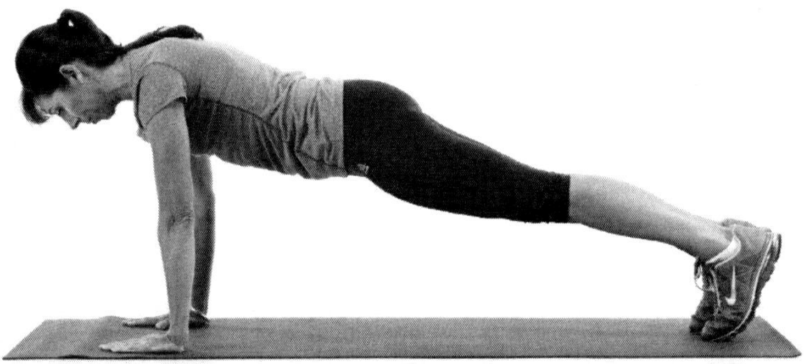

Abdominal Muscle Strength Training Equipment

Some high resistance abdominal exercise machines have the potential to increase pressure within the abdomen and overload the pelvic floor. Women with poorly functioning pelvic floor muscles and those having undergone prolapse surgery can reduce the load on their pelvic floor by using minimal resistance or avoiding these machines altogether. The following list of abdominal exercise equipment includes examples of the types of equipment requiring caution if you have a prolapse.

Abdominal exercise equipment requiring caution:

- Spring loaded abdominal resistance machines (e.g. Pilates reformer high resistance abdominal muscle exercises)
- Abdominal crunch plate-loaded resistance machines (e.g. seated abdominal crunch gym machine)
- Abdominal crunch hydraulic circuit equipment
- Abdominal rolling out exercise devices
- Abdominal crunch frames

How to Modify Intense Core Abdominal Exercises

The intensity of core abdominal exercises can often be modified to reduce pressure on the pelvic floor. Some women with poor pelvic floor support may need to avoid intense core exercises altogether (e.g. after prolapse surgery or with weak pelvic floor muscles) and instead choose the pelvic floor safe abdominal core exercises (Chapter 5). Other women find they can perform modified abdominal exercises as their pelvic floor muscle support improves with pelvic floor rehabilitation.

The level of intensity of your abdominal exercises is largely dependent upon the level of support your pelvic floor provides for your pelvic organs. If you are not sure about how well your pelvic floor muscles are working, a pelvic floor physiotherapy assessment can provide you with this information.

Guide to Modifying Intense Core Abdominal Exercises

This guide helps you understand how to modify intense abdominal exercises to reduce the load on your pelvic floor with abdominal exercises.

1. ***Breathe out with the effort***
Avoid holding your breath during abdominal exercises and try to breathe out as your abdominal muscles contract.

2. ***Never strain***
Abdominal exercises that cause you to strain are too intense - always keep your abdominal exercises at a manageable level of intensity.

3. ***Avoid intense abdominal muscle bracing***
Brace or contract your abdominal muscles gently using the abdominal activation technique outlined in Chapter 5. Strong abdominal bracing is inappropriate with prolapse problems.

4. ***Minimise the number of repetitions***
Avoid overloading your pelvic floor with too many repeated abdominal exercises. Gradually progress your abdominal exercises keeping the number of exercises you perform within a manageable range.

5. ***Modify double leg raise exercises***
Avoid double leg raises and modify by raising only one leg at a time, keeping your head and shoulders down in contact with the supporting surface throughout.

6. ***Reduce the load supported by your upper limbs***
Upper body weight bearing exercises can increase the load on your pelvic floor. Reduce this load by decreasing the amount of weight supported through your forearms or hands. Intense core exercises such as plank, hover or men's push ups can be modified by kneeling weight bearing through the feet. Wall push ups can be modified by moving your feet closer to the wall.

7. ***Minimise the resistance of abdominal machines***
Abdominal exercise machines often have adjustable load or resistance. Adjust the level of resistance to keep the exercise intensity manageable for your pelvic floor.

Key Points for Abdominal Exercises and Prolapse

- Some mainstream intense core abdominal strength exercises are inappropriate for women with, or at risk of prolapse problems.
- Knowing how to identify and modify unsafe abdominal strength exercises is important for women with prolapse problems.
- The pelvic floor and abdominal muscles should work together in a balanced and coordinated manner.
- Two main pelvic floor problems can be caused by intense abdominal core exercises: pelvic floor overload or pelvic floor overbracing.
- Pelvic floor overload occurs when the pelvic floor is unable to withstand the pressure generated by intense abdominal muscle exercises.
- Pelvic floor overbracing occurs with intense core exercise and insufficient pelvic floor muscle relaxation.
- Intense abdominal core exercises can contribute to pelvic floor strain and weakness in some women with pelvic floor dysfunction.
- The intensity of your core abdominal muscle exercises should match the level of support provided by your pelvic floor.
- Core exercises most likely to overload the pelvic floor are intense upper abdominal strength exercises.
- Intense abdominal muscle exercises include head and trunk raises, double leg raises, weight bearing through the upper limbs and abdominal resistance training equipment.
- Some intense abdominal core exercises can be modified to reduce the intensity and associated pelvic floor loading.

7 Aerobic Fitness Exercises and Prolapse

Fitness exercises are also known as aerobic or cardiorespiratory exercises. These exercises noticeably increase heart rate and promote heart and lung fitness. If you avoid or limit aerobic fitness exercises because of your prolapse, this can have a negative effect upon your overall health and well being. Women with prolapse can often continue to perform appropriate aerobic fitness exercises and reap the associated health benefits without worsening their prolapse problems.

Benefits of Fitness Exercise for Women

There are substantial health benefits to be gained by women who participate in regular aerobic fitness exercise. With menopause, women lose the protective effects of oestrogen so that the risk of some chronic diseases increases. Women can decrease their risk of some specific chronic health diseases and improve their overall health and wellbeing through participation in regular aerobic fitness exercise.

Benefits of aerobic fitness exercise include:

- Decreased risk of heart disease, stroke, Type 2 diabetes and some forms of cancer (e.g. breast cancer, colon cancer).
- Improved energy levels, weight management, sleep, mood, mental health and sense of wellbeing.

Exercise Selection and Prolapse

If you have been diagnosed with a prolapse, it is important that you understand the potential risks with high impact fitness exercises. High impact exercises involve landing heavily, usually after having both feet off the ground at once. High impact exercises increase the load on the pelvic floor with landing. The greater the impact of landing or with repeated landing impact, the greater the potential to overload and weaken internal pelvic floor supports.

The risk of overloading the pelvic floor with high impact exercise increases with:

- Excess abdominal body fat
- Poor pelvic floor support
- Previous pelvic prolapse surgery

Some women mistakenly believe that after having their prolapse repaired they can safely return to high impact exercises. After prolapse surgery, the pelvic floor organs are at increased risk of repeat prolapse and high impact exercises should usually be avoided.

Pelvic floor safe fitness exercises are low impact exercises. Low impact exercise minimises the impact of the landing forces on the pelvic floor. Exercises are low impact when at least one foot remains in contact with the supporting surface at all times. Alternatively, exercises where the body weight is supported are also low impact, for example cycling or swimming. Low impact fitness exercises generally allow women to exercise effectively for their aerobic fitness while placing minimal strain on the pelvic floor.

Pelvic Floor Safe Low Impact Exercises

Low impact exercises are the most appropriate fitness exercises for women with prolapse problems. The following exercises are low impact and more appropriate for women with prolapse than high impact exercises:

- Walking
- Hiking
- Cycling
- Low impact dancing
- Low impact fitness classes

- Step exercise (low height step)
- Elliptical machine (low resistance)
- Swimming
- Water walking
- Kayaking
- Cross country skiing (gentle downward slope)
- Social tennis

High Impact Fitness Exercises to Avoid

High impact exercises have the potential to overload the pelvic floor and are best avoided by most women with prolapse problems.

Aerobic fitness exercises that involve high impact landing include:

- Running
- Jumping
- Hopping
- Skipping
- Star jumps
- Burpees
- Step exercises (jumping off step)
- High box step downs
- Plyometric jumping exercises
- High impact exercise classes
- Netball
- Basketball
- Volleyball

Tips to modify impact exercises

To reduce the impact of some high impact exercises:

- Walk briskly and swing your arms rather than run
- Vary walking surfaces
- Reduce stepping height
- Choose low impact alternatives e.g. mini squats rather than jumps, side steps rather than star jumps
- Include supported exercises e.g. cycling
- Vary your low impact exercises regularly

Aerobic Fitness Exercise Guidelines for Healthy Women

The recommended quantity of exercise for achieving cardiovascular fitness in healthy adults:[10]

- At least 30 minutes of moderate intensity aerobic exercise on 5 days or more (total at least 150 minutes or 2.5 hrs/week)

or

- At least 20 minutes of high intensity aerobic exercise on 3 days or more (total at least 75 minutes or 1.25 hrs/week)

plus

- Exercise sessions can be made up of short sessions of at least 10 minutes duration or one continuous longer session
- Even if you are unable to meet these minimum requirements you will still benefit from some physical aerobic activity
- Regularly progress the quantity of aerobic fitness exercise you perform as your fitness improves over time.

Key Points for Aerobic Fitness Exercises for Prolapse

- ♀ Aerobic exercise is another term for cardiorespiratory fitness exercise.
- ♀ Aerobic fitness exercise improves heart and lung health.
- ♀ Aerobic exercise involves physical activity that noticeably increases your heart rate.
- ♀ Aerobic fitness exercise has numerous physical and emotional benefits for women.
- ♀ Many women with prolapse can continue to exercise for fitness without worsening their prolapse.
- ♀ High impact exercises are those that generate high forces when the feet strike the ground.
- ♀ Some high impact exercises pose more risk to some women than others, owing to individual differences.
- ♀ Low impact exercises minimise pelvic floor loading when compared with high impact aerobic exercises.
- ♀ Low impact exercises provide a pelvic floor safe aerobic fitness alternative for women with prolapse.
- ♀ Modify the impact of high impact exercises where feasible if you have prolapse problems.
- ♀ Aim to perform at least 30 minutes of moderate intensity low impact exercise for fitness on at least 5 days of the week.
- ♀ If you are able to exercise at high intensity, aim to perform at least 20 minutes of vigorous intensity, low impact exercise on at least 3 days of the week.

Section III

Exercises for Prolapse & Special Health Needs

8 Exercise After Prolapse Surgery

Exercise after prolapse surgery can reduce post-operative risks and promote physical recovery. This chapter provides information about two types of post-operative exercises that may be recommended by your physiotherapist: exercises for early post-operative recovery and exercises generally suited to the 6 weeks after surgery.

Recovery exercises after prolapse surgery aim to:

1. Prevent and minimise some of the risks and side effects of prolapse surgery.
2. Minimise the physical decline that occurs with bed rest and decreased mobility, especially during the first 6-8 weeks after surgery.

> Exercise during the early stages of prolapse surgery recovery is never directed at improving fitness or weight loss.

Early Post-operative Recovery

Early recovery exercises are directed towards reducing some of the potential risks associated with prolapse surgery. Post-operative exercises are usually guided by physiotherapy and/or nursing staff during the hospital stay. The following exercises are intended as general information about post-operative prolapse repair exercises. Post-operative exercises can vary according to a woman's risk factors, pre-existing general health conditions as well as post-operative problems should they occur.

Deep Breathing Exercises

Deep breathing exercises are usually encouraged immediately after surgery. Deep breathing improves circulating oxygen levels and minimises the risk of post-operative chest complications. You may be encouraged to take some deep breaths by your nurse when you first wake after surgery. Most women are usually encouraged to do 4-5 deep breaths every hour during waking hours, particularly when confined to bed, however this can vary according to individual risks or post-operative chest problems.

Deep breathing involves a technique called diaphragmatic breathing. If you have ever done Yoga breathing you may already be familiar with this breathing technique. Diaphragmatic breathing can be practised by placing your hands just above your waist on the lower margins of your rib cage. You should be able to feel your waist widen beneath your hands as you slowly breathe in and fill your lungs with air. You should notice your hands move outwards and your upper abdomen move forwards as you breathe in. Gently relax your chest wall to breathe out and notice your waist narrow and your rib cage move back to resting position.

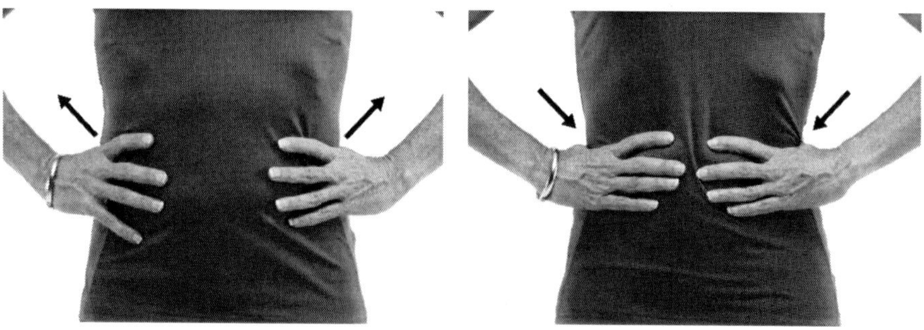

a. Breathe in - waist widens b. Breathe out - waist narrows

After surgery, the first few deep breaths can sometimes make you feel as though you need to cough, however deep breathing should not be avoided for this reason. There are some useful strategies you can use to help you reduce discomfort and pressure on your pelvic floor if you need to cough after surgery.

How to manage coughing:

1. Place your hand outside your briefs, over your sanitary pad, to provide some external support to your pelvic floor if you feel the need to cough.

2. Use 'The Knack' exercise technique described in Chapter 2 to gently lift your pelvic floor muscles prior to and during a cough.

3. If you have a chronic chest complaint that causes you to cough, discuss appropriate post-operative medication with your doctor prior to your surgery.

Circulation Exercises

Circulation exercises aim to reduce the risk of blood clots forming in the deep veins of the legs after surgery. These blood clots are known as deep vein thrombosis (DVT).

Circulation exercises are simple exercises that promote blood flow in the deep veins of the lower body to reduce the risk of blood clots forming in these veins. You may have been encouraged to do similar circulation exercises to prevent DVT during long plane flights.

Circulation exercises performed regularly when resting in bed:

- *Calf pumps* - bend and straighten your ankles to gently move your feet up and down 10 times in a row, keeping your legs straight throughout (shown over page).
- *Thigh muscle squeezes* - contract your thigh muscles with your legs outstretched by gently pressing the back of your

knees into the bed. Squeeze your thigh muscles for 5 seconds at a time and then relax back to resting.

- *Buttock squeezes* - gently squeeze your buttocks while lying down, maintain this squeeze for 5 seconds at a time and then relax your buttock muscles back to resting.

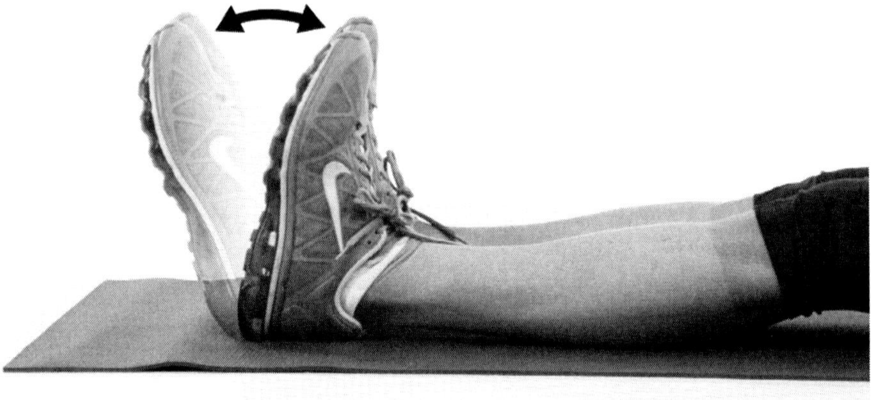

Post-operative Walking

There are numerous benefits to be gained from early mobilisation (movement) after prolapse surgery. Getting out of bed and walking encourages physical recovery and prevents chest and circulation problems associated with prolonged bed rest. Walking promotes bowel movement and alleviates joint pain, including neck and back pain that can occur with bed rest. Most women usually report feeling much better having moved out of bed, despite the fact that it can initially seem daunting.

Walking after surgery commences upon your surgeon's direction. Some women commence walking on the day following surgery, while others may require longer recovery time in bed. You can usually expect to be assisted into sitting with your legs over the side of the bed by the nurse or physiotherapist before standing up. Your first steps may involve walking on the spot or walking a short distance to the bathroom, or in the hospital corridor. You can expect to be accompanied during walking until you are considered safe to walk on your own. The time spent walking is usually progressed gradually during your hospital stay. Most women are able to comfortably walk short distances without assistance upon discharge from hospital.

Tips for early post-operative walking

- Avoid standing up too quickly after sitting or lying down. Some women feel lightheaded or wobbly on their feet when they stand up after surgery. Sit briefly with your legs over the side of the bed before standing up.
- Standing up and walking can sometimes trigger the urge to empty the bladder or bowel. Anticipate when you may next need to visit the bathroom to avoid being caught by surprise and needing to rush.
- Ask someone to accompany you during walking if you feel at all unsteady or unsure of your balance after surgery.
- Ask for a chair to be positioned in close proximity to your bed, should you need to sit down quickly.
- Wear well fitting slippers rather than loose scuffs to avoid tripping when walking.

Bed Recovery Exercises

Some basic exercises can help to alleviate joint stiffness and allow for safe movement when resting in bed. Be guided by your treating physiotherapist regarding the exercises that are most appropriate for your recovery and how often to repeat them. Post-operative exercises should never cause physical discomfort.

Sample Bed Recovery Exercises

Heel Slides

Heel slides promote circulation and can help to alleviate knee, hip or lower back stiffness.

Starting position: Lying on your back with your legs out straight.

Action: Slide one heel along the bed towards your bottom by bending your knee, and then slide your heel back to starting position.

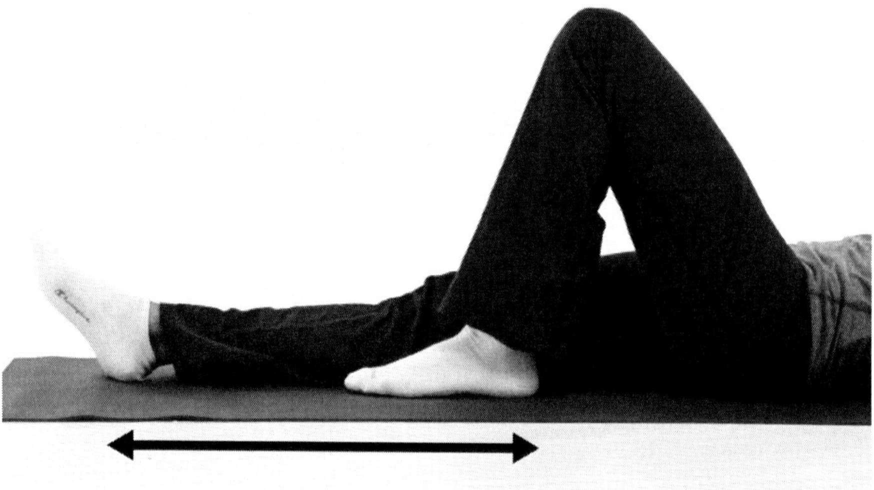

Knee Rolls

Knee rolls can help to avoid or overcome stiffness in the lower back.

Starting position: Lying on your back with your knees bent and feet flat on the bed.

Action: Keep your knees close together and lower both knees slightly towards the mattress on one side of your body. Return back to your starting position and repeat to the other side. This is a small rolling movement and does not involve twisting too far through your trunk. Avoid lowering your knees right down to the mattress, particularly if you have an abdominal wound.

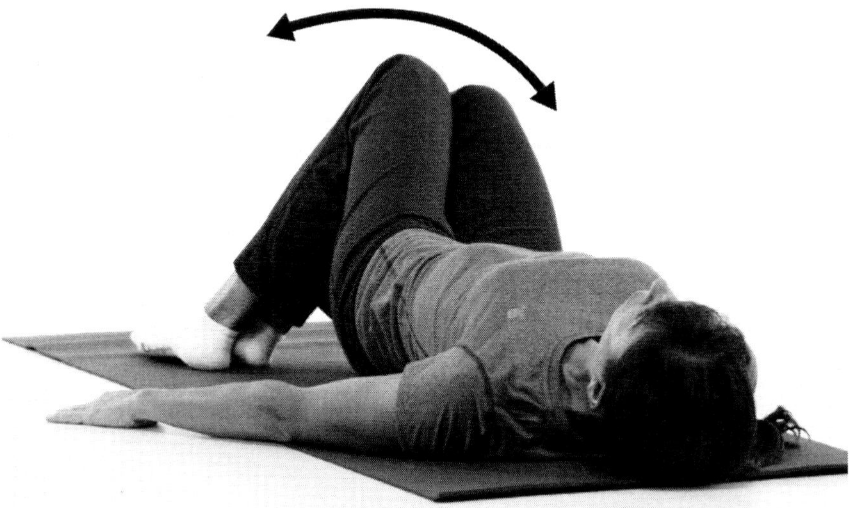

Pelvic Tilts

Pelvic tilts can help avoid and alleviate lower back stiffness and discomfort.

Starting position: Lying on your back with your knees bent and feet flat on the bed. You should be aware of a light inward curve in your lower back.

Action: Gently flatten the inward curve in your lower back by tilting or rolling your pelvis backwards. Release and roll your pelvis back to your starting position and repeat.

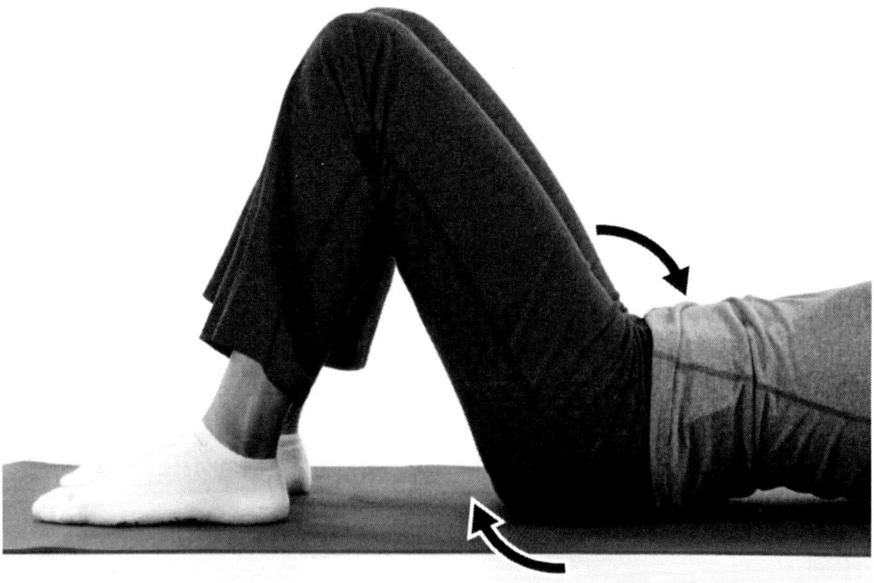

Bridges

Bridges can help you to move with minimal discomfort and relieve pressure off the buttocks and lower back. Bridging is a useful technique for moving in bed using your buttocks instead of your abdominal muscles to minimise pressure on the pelvic floor as you move.

Starting position: Lying on your back with your knees bent and feet flat on the bed.

Action: Push down through your heels to slightly raise your buttocks to a comfortable height off the bed. Lower your buttocks back to the bed and repeat this action.

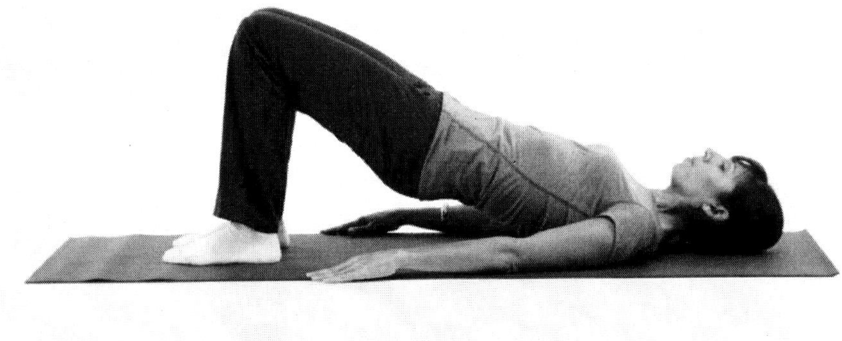

Exercises After Hospital Discharge

Walking is the exercise of choice for most women during post-operative recovery. Walking is a low impact, whole body exercise that can be gradually progressed. Women usually benefit from a combination of bed recovery exercises and walking exercises during the first 6 weeks after discharge from hospital.

Walking promotes physical and emotional recovery from prolapse surgery. Regular walking after surgery can help to:

- Minimise physical deterioration in strength and fitness
- Prevent and relieve joint pain and stiffness
- Minimise the risk of post-operative chest problems
- Improve circulation which reduces the risk of blood clots
- Improve gut motility to promote bowel movement and alleviate wind (gas) discomfort
- Improve feelings of wellbeing and reduce feelings of stress or anxiety.

Walking Guidelines After Prolapse Repair

1. Commence your home walking program only with your surgeon's approval.
2. Listen to your body and aim to maintain a manageable level of physical comfort during and after walking. Pain or undue discomfort associated with walking can be an indication that you are doing too much, too soon.
3. Walk at your own pace.
4. Progress your walking program gradually as your body heals.
5. Walk when you feel rested, rather than when you are fatigued.
6. Balance your walking exercise with sufficient rest so that you put your feet up and rest after walking.
7. Time your walking exercise to coincide with adequate pain relief medication.
8. Contact your surgeon with any concerns you may encounter regarding your post-operative walking exercise.

General Guide for Walking

Women differ in terms of how much walking they can do after prolapse surgery - there is no one rule fits all. This walking guide outlines the level of walking that most women can comfortably achieve during their early recovery after discharge from hospital. It can be useful to use a time-based approach to your walking program so that you can readily monitor and progress the time you spend walking during your recovery.

Your individual walking program is determined by your surgeon's guidelines for you. This information is intended as a general guide for the amount of walking you might expect as you recover at home.

Weeks 1-2

Most women are encouraged to continue their in-hospital walking routine when first discharged. This typically involves short 5-10 minute walks that are repeated at intervals throughout the day. By the end of the second week, women can usually walk continuously for up to 10 minutes at a time.

Weeks 3-4

It is usually appropriate to aim to increase the total time spent walking daily, by approximately 5 minutes per week. In keeping with this formula, by the end of week 4 many women are able to walk for 20 minutes without stopping. An ideal alternative to a longer duration walk is to opt for a couple of shorter duration, 10 minute walks throughout the day.

Weeks 5-6

By the end of week 6, many women can comfortably walk for 30 minutes continuously. Women who are unable to do long continuous walks will benefit from doing 2-3 shorter, 10 minute walks throughout the day.

Week 7 onwards

Most women have a check up with their specialist at around 6 weeks after prolapse surgery. At this appointment your doctor may discuss your exercise program and give you permission to proceed towards returning to your regular exercise routine. If you have permission to progress your walking program, then this is the time you may start to increase your walking speed.

Be mindful of the fact that while you may appear to be healed from the outside, your internal wound will continue to heal for up to 3 months after your surgery. During this time it is important to gradually progress your walking program so as to avoid undue strain on your repair.

Treadmill Walking After Surgery

Walking on a treadmill differs to walking outdoors. Walking outside involves natural changes in pace and surface variations. Walking on a treadmill is more demanding than walking outdoors as the pace is dictated by the walking machine. If you intend to walk on a treadmill after surgery, hold onto the side bars with your hands when you start out, keep the gradient flat and progress at a slower rate than walking outdoors. Be mindful of the potential for your balance to be temporarily decreased after surgery. Commence treadmill walking only when you are completely sure of your balance and stability.

Tips for Home-Based Walking Exercise

- Try to walk with tall posture
- Wear well fitting cushioned footwear
- Short frequent walks are an excellent alternative to long continuous walks
- Progress the time you spend walking rather than the distance
- Choose flat surfaces and avoid hills where possible
- Avoid walking when you are fatigued
- Rest after walking, ideally lying down to relieve the load on your pelvic floor
- Quality support briefs or bike pants can sometimes improve comfort when walking
- Avoid walking your dog on a lead to avoid potential strain to your repair

Key Points for Exercise After Prolapse Surgery

- ♀ Initial exercise after prolapse surgery is directed at reducing potential risks, side effects and minimising physical deterioration.
- ♀ Exercises to reduce some post-operative risks include deep breathing exercises, circulation exercises and early mobilisation out of bed.
- ♀ Walking is usually commenced in the early days after prolapse surgery to promote physical recovery.
- ♀ Recovery exercises performed in bed may help to relieve joint stiffness, physical discomfort and increase circulation.
- ♀ Walking is the exercise of choice after prolapse surgery for most women and there are numerous physical and emotional benefits to be gained.
- ♀ Commence walking at home only with your surgeon's approval.
- ♀ Walking after prolapse surgery should be: comfortable, gradually progressed, self paced, progressed according to the time spent walking, timed to coincide with adequate pain relief and balanced with adequate rest.
- ♀ It is usually appropriate to aim to progress daily walking by 5 minutes per week.
- ♀ Most women can perform 30 minutes of continuous walking at around 6 weeks after prolapse surgery.
- ♀ Treadmill walking is more challenging than walking outdoors and requires good balance and stability.

9 Osteoporosis Exercises and Prolapse

Osteoporosis is a condition where bones become fragile, brittle and prone to fracture. In women the natural decline in bone density starts at around forty years of age, with bone loss accelerating rapidly in the years immediately following menopause. Menopause is also when many women notice a worsening of their pelvic floor problems, including pelvic organ prolapse. Both osteoporosis and pelvic organ prolapse can be affected by menopausal hormonal changes.

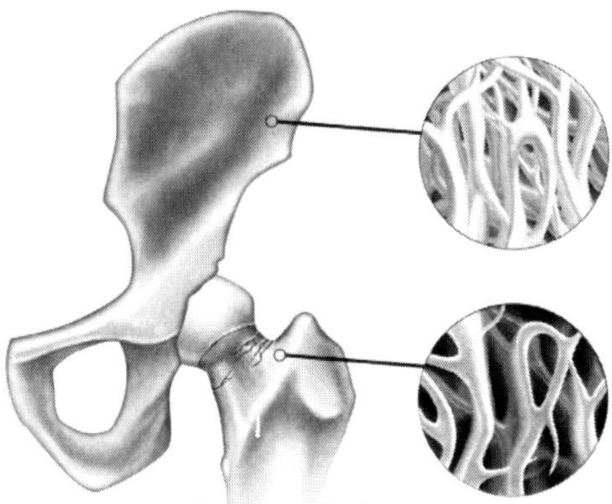

Osteoporotic Bone

Osteoporosis can impact upon a woman's pelvic floor health. Middle aged and elderly women with osteoporosis are at increased risk of developing pelvic organ prolapse.[12] The slumped forwards posture that results from decreased spinal bone density and spinal fractures increases downward pressure upon the pelvic floor. The pelvic floor muscles work less effectively when the spine is slumped forwards. The loss of height associated with osteoporosis is also associated with increased urinary incontinence in elderly women.[13]

Pelvic organ prolapse may impact indirectly upon a woman's bone health. Women with prolapse may be less inclined to perform bone health exercises for fear of worsening their condition or aggravating their prolapse symptoms. As a result some women miss out on the potential benefits of exercise for their bone health. This is often unnecessary since in many cases women with pelvic prolapse can exercise effectively for their bone health and protect their pelvic floor.

Bone Density Exercises

Exercise is an important factor in preventing and managing osteoporosis. Bone density exercises improve bone health by loading or applying forces to bones. Bones are living tissue and when they are loaded with appropriate forces, they can respond with improved bone density and structural changes.[14]

The two main types of exercise prescribed to improve bone density are weight bearing exercise and strength training exercises.

1. *Weight Bearing Exercise*

Weight bearing exercise for bone density involves impact exercise that is performed supporting the body weight mostly through the feet.

2. *Strength Training Exercises*

Strength training exercise for bone density involves using specific muscle groups against the force of a load.

Bone Density Exercise and Prolapse

Osteoporosis exercise presents a unique challenge for women with pelvic organ prolapse. High impact exercise and heavily loaded strength training exercises known to most effectively improve bone density also have the potential to overload the pelvic floor. Unfortunately both these types of exercise are associated with intense physical forces that are usually unsuitable for women with prolapse problems. These exercises are also unsuitable for many women with osteoporosis owing to the increased fracture risk associated with high impact and heavily loaded resistance exercises.

If you have prolapse problems and decreased bone density it's important to understand the potential for inappropriate bone health exercises to worsen prolapse symptoms or cause pelvic floor injury after prolapse surgery.

Bone Health Exercise Program

A complete bone health exercise program should incorporate exercises for posture, muscle strength, fitness and flexibility. These exercises can usually be modified for women with prolapse problems.

Combine the following exercises in your complete bone health exercise program:

- Posture exercises
    - improve posture, reduce the strain on the spine and reduce the risk of falling. Falls are often the cause of bone fractures with osteoporosis.
- Muscle strength exercises
    - strengthen bones, muscles, and reduce the risk of falls.
- Balance exercises
    - reduce the risk of falls and address the natural decline in balance with increasing age.
- Fitness exercises
    - improve cardiovascular fitness, stamina and weight management.
- Flexibility exercises
    - promote good posture, reduce spinal joint stiffness and discomfort, decrease the risk of falls.

Bone Health Exercises for Caution

Mature women sometimes commence bone health exercise programs and find they develop or worsen their pelvic floor problems as a result. Some specific bone density exercises require caution to reduce the risk of prolapse problems developing or worsening.

1. *High Impact Exercises*

High impact exercises involve forceful rapid loading of the bones with exercises involving both feet off the ground at once and landing forcefully. These exercises effectively load bones to promote new bone formation, however they also load the pelvic floor and are not appropriate for most women with prolapse or with increased risk of pelvic floor injury. High impact exercises are also inappropriate for women with established osteoporosis owing to the increased risk of fracture with these exercises.

High impact exercises to avoid with prolapse and osteoporosis include:

- Running
- Jumping
- Skipping
- Jumping up and down stairs

2. *High Force Resistance Exercises*

High force, heavily loaded resistance exercises, load bones to promote bone formation. Resistance exercise for bone loading typically involves high resistance or heavy loads that are progressed over time. High resistance bone loading exercises often involve near maximum voluntary effort against the load with a low number of repeated exercises or repetitions. Heavy load resistance training has the potential to cause women at risk of pelvic floor problems to strain and overload their pelvic floor, or risk osteoporotic fracture in women with established osteoporosis.

Pelvic Floor Safe Bone Health Exercises

In women with increased risk of pelvic organ prolapse, the focus of bone health exercise shifts from heavy impact bone loading, to a modified exercise approach with exercises designed to promote bone health and prevent or minimise the decline in bone density with increasing age.

The following exercises are designed to improve your understanding about appropriate bone health exercises with a prolapse. These sample exercises and modifications are intended as general information. If you have established osteoporosis seek your doctor's approval before commencing any new exercise program. Supervised and individualised exercise programs are most desirable for women with established osteoporosis or osteoporotic fractures.

Posture Exercises

1. Posture Correction Exercise

Posture correction helps to reduce strain on the spine and associated discomfort. Posture exercises can also reduce the load on the pelvic floor by decreasing pressure within the abdomen and allowing the pelvic floor muscles to work more effectively.

Start

Sit or stand side on to a mirror and look at your posture. Typically with osteoporosis the upper middle back is rounded forwards. You may notice your upper back slumped, shoulders rolled forwards and chin poking outwards.

Action

- Lift your chest or breast bone forwards and upwards
- Lift the crown of your head towards the ceiling to lengthen your spine
- Relax your neck and shoulders
- Avoid overarching your lower back

Result

Your mid spine should appear less rounded, your shoulders should roll back and your neck should poke less. Ideally you should see an inward curve in your lower back however this can be difficult if you have spinal fractures.

Posture Correction

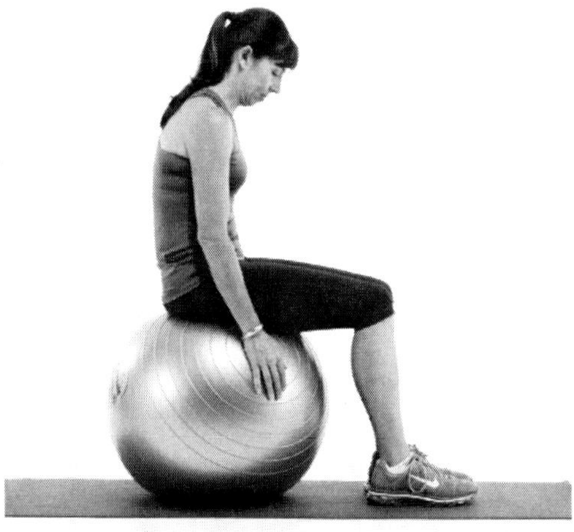

Slumped forwards

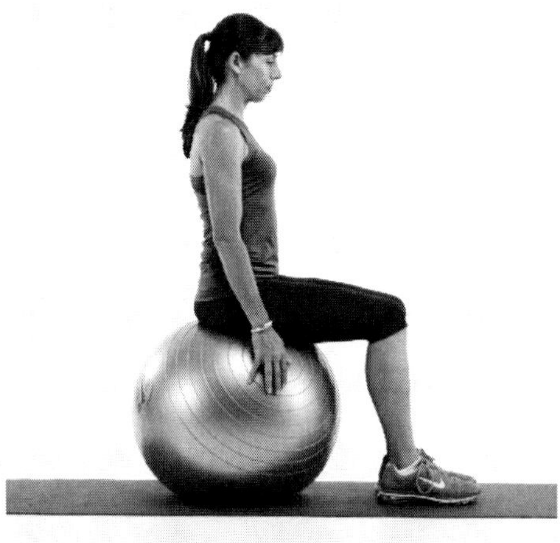

Posture corrected

2. *Shoulder Blade Squeeze*

Start

Sit or stand holding an exercise band in both of your hands, elbows tucked into your waist, palms facing the ceiling and thumbs turned outwards.

Action

Stretch the resistance band by moving one or both of your forearms outwards in opposite directions, keeping your elbows tucked into your waist throughout. When you reach your limit of outward movement, slowly return back to your starting position. Repeat up to 8-12 times, then repeat the set again. Aim for the 2 sets to be done on 3 alternate week days.

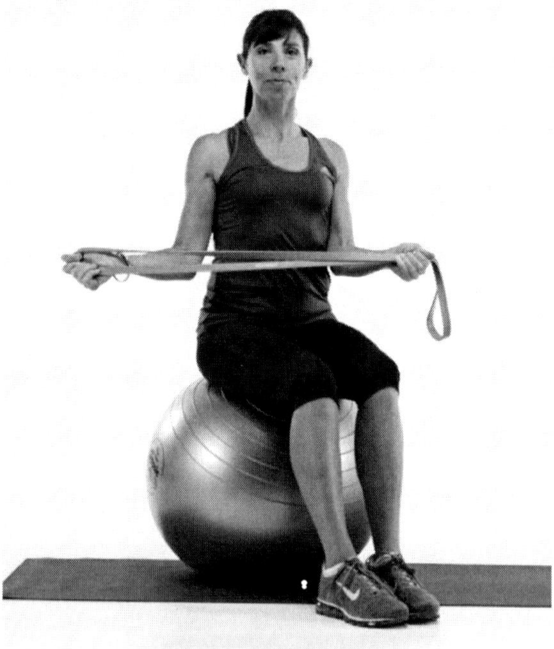

Shoulder Blade Squeeze moving one forearm

3. *Push Backs*

Start

Kneel, or lay prone with your arms extended beside your trunk and palms facing downwards or towards the sides of your body. If you are prone to lower back pain, place a pillow or cushion under your hips and pelvis before commencing this exercise to reduce strain on your spine.

Action

Raise both arms backwards keeping your arms extended and squeeze your shoulder blades together. Slowly lower your arms and return your arms back to your sides. Progress this exercise with dumb-bell weights as shown below. Repeat up to 8-12 times, then repeat the set again. Aim for the 2 sets to be done on 3 alternate week days.

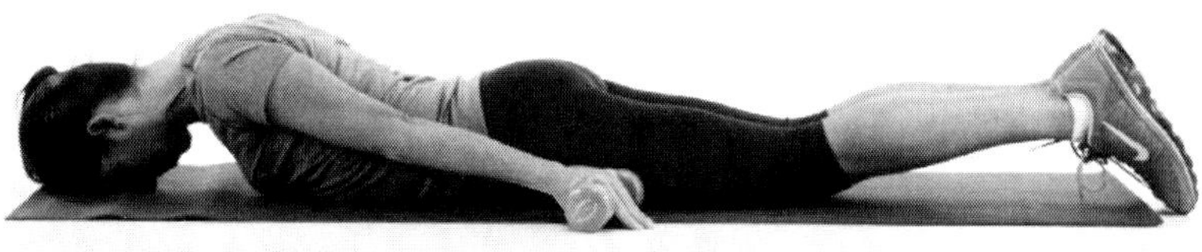

Push Backs a. starting position

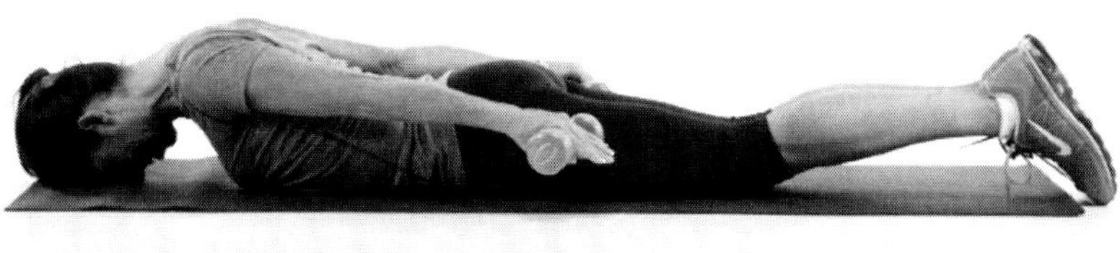

Push Backs b. action

Muscle Strength Exercises

The goal of muscle strength exercises for bone health is to load those bones at greatest risk of fracture: the hips, spine and wrists. Bone loading with resistance exercise occurs via the direct muscle pull on the bones. If the stimulus for bone formation is sufficient, this pull promotes the production of new bone cells where the muscle attaches to the bone. In this way, bone formation is specific to the muscles being exercised. For example if your hip bone density is decreased, the best bone loading exercises are those that strengthen the hip and buttock muscles that attach close to your hip bones. Upper body exercises won't improve your hip bone density.

In women with osteoporosis and pelvic organ prolapse, the focus shifts away from high load, low repetition resistance bone density exercise. Instead the emphasis is upon light to moderate intensity resistance exercises that are progressed over time with improved pelvic floor strength and control.

The following muscle strength exercises are examples of those usually appropriate for inclusion into pelvic floor safe bone health exercise programs:

1. *Leg and hip exercises*
    - Mini squats*
    - Hip extension prone
    - Hamstring curl
    - Bridge supine*
    - Clam side lying
    - Calf raises*

2. *Trunk exercises*
    - Prone trunk extension
    - Seated row
    - Kneeling or lying prone alternate arm raise - progress to alternate arm and leg raises*

3. *Arm and chest exercises*

- Standing wall push ups
- Biceps curl with wrist rotation*
- Triceps extension*
- Overhead dumbbell press

* Exercises described in Chapter 4 and demonstrated in Pelvic Exercises Strength DVD.[8]

Pelvic Floor Safe Muscle Strength Exercise Dosage for Bone Health

- Use light - moderate resistance loading
- Include 8-10 exercises for the muscle groups listed above
- Build up to 2-4 sets (groups) of 8-12 repetitions (repeated exercises)
- Perform strength exercises on 2-3 times a week on alternate days
- Gradually progress the amount of exercise you perform over time
- Employ those guidelines outlined in the 10 Step Guide to Pelvic Floor Safe Strength Training for Prolapse (Chapter 4)

Balance Exercises

Most of us take our balance for granted, without recognising the benefits of specific balance exercises with increasing age. Balance training aims to reduce the risk of falls and is therefore an essential component of bone health exercise. There are numerous balance exercises that are readily performed and progressed to promote better balance. Balance exercises are usually pelvic floor safe exercises and therefore appropriate for women with pelvic organ prolapse.

Standing balance exercises

Balance exercises are ideally performed on a daily basis for 10-15 minutes, prior to doing strength exercises so that the muscles are rested rather than fatigued. Practice your balance exercises near a firm support such as a wall or fixed bench to reduce your risk of falling, especially if you have poor balance.

Sample balance exercises include:

- Standing with one foot in front of the other
- Standing on one leg
- Standing heel to toe raises
- Heel to toe walking
- Tai Chi is known to reduce the risk of falls in older adults and is a gentle low impact pelvic floor safe exercise

Progressing balance exercises

Balance training should be progressed gradually as balance improves. Balance exercises are readily progressed with the use of balance training equipment and by altering some specific elements of balance exercises. There are many ways to progress balance exercises, for example:

- Increase the instability of the supporting surface (e.g. upper body strength exercises whilst sitting on a chair progressing to exercises sitting on an exercise ball)
- Decrease the visual input (e.g. balance exercises performed with eyes open progressing to eyes closed)
- Reduce upper body support during exercises (e.g. balance exercises holding the wall with both hands progressing to holding with one hand, and then no hands)

Fitness Exercises

High impact fitness exercises are usually advocated for promoting bone formation. While high impact exercises are known to be most effective for bone loading, they are inappropriate for women with, or at risk of pelvic organ prolapse (see Chapter 7), as well as women with high fracture risk.

Low impact exercises are the most appropriate fitness exercises for women with prolapse and osteoporosis. Appropriate low impact exercise promotes cardiovascular fitness, stamina and weight management. As outlined in Chapter 7, low impact exercise minimises the load on the pelvic floor when compared with high impact exercise.

Pelvic floor safe low impact fitness exercises include:

- Brisk walking
- Cycling
- Swimming
- Low impact dancing

Walking and bone density

Walking is an excellent low impact exercise for many women with prolapse and osteoporosis, however walking is not the exercise of choice for improving bone density. Unfortunately slow walking exercise will not improve bone density, perhaps owing to the fact that it is a regular everyday activity which the bones are usually well-accustomed to doing. Aim to walk briskly where possible, since walking exercise needs to be very brisk to increase bone density. Carrying dumbbell weights is never advisable with walking as it can increase the potential for injury. Some women choose to perform walking exercise wearing weighted vests however women with pelvic organ prolapse need to remember that the added weight in the vest will also increase the load on their pelvic floor when they walk.

Flexibility Exercises

With osteoporosis some of the joints and muscles of the body become less flexible. Flexibility exercises can promote good posture and alleviate joint stiffness. Flexibility exercises should be directed at specific areas of the body to promote improved posture, spinal joint mobility and ability to walk without falling.

There are numerous flexibility exercises for bone health and osteoporosis and a comprehensive list is beyond the scope of this book. Sample pelvic floor safe flexibility exercises for osteoporosis include:

1. *Calf muscle stretch*

Calf stretching is designed to reduce the risk of falling associated with tight shortened calf muscles.

Starting position

Lean against a wall with your hands at approximately shoulder height or above. Position your legs in a forward lunge position with one leg forward and the other leg extended behind your body.

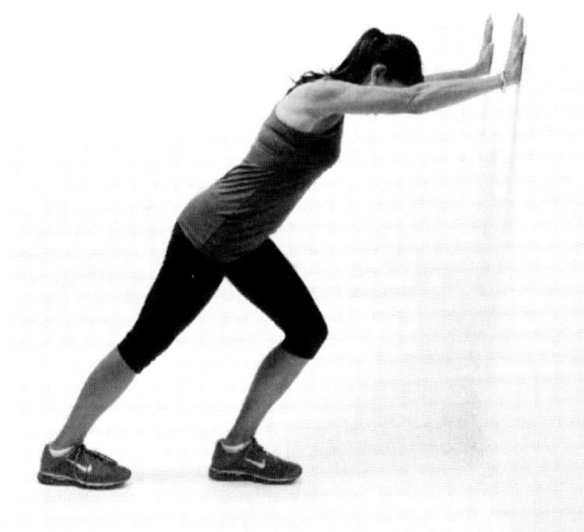

Action

Lower your back heel to the ground and straighten out your back knee to stretch the calf muscle in your back leg. If you are unable to feel the calf stretch, step your back foot further backwards. Perform this exercise for at least 10-30 seconds, repeat 3 times daily.

2. *Corner chest stretch*

Chest stretching exercises can help promote good upright posture and reduce slumped forwards posture.

Starting position

Face a corner where two walls meet, with your forearms placed on or close to the walls, elbows approximately shoulder height and standing in a forward lunge position.

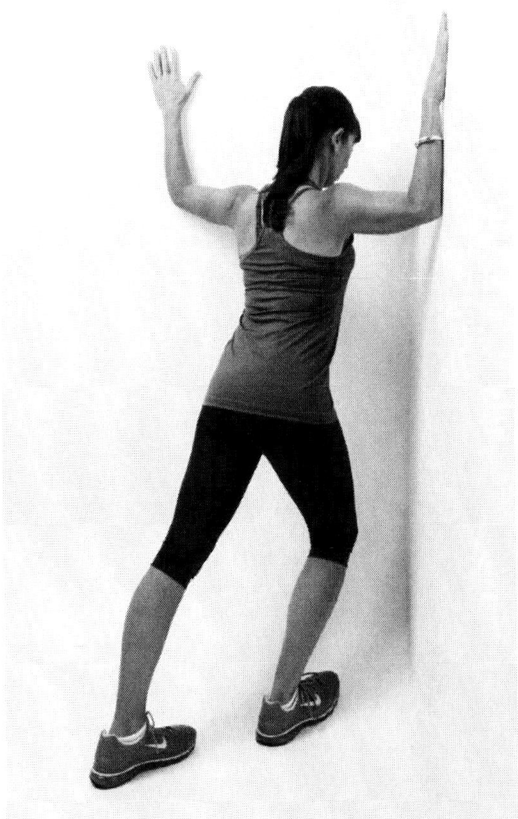

Action

Lean your chest forwards towards the corner - you should feel a gentle stretch across your chest and front of shoulders. Maintain this position for at least 10-30 seconds, repeat 3 times daily.

Tip

If you are prone to shoulder discomfort, you may find that stretching one side of your chest at a time or lowering the height of your elbows against the wall may feel more comfortable.

3. *Mid spine mobility exercise*

Mid spine rotation aims to improve movement and alleviate middle spine stiffness.

Starting position

Sit facing forwards with your finger tips resting on your shoulders.

Action

Slowly and gently turn your body to rotate your trunk in one direction and then in the opposite direction. Try to breathe out as you rotate your body to the side. Repeat daily, 5 times each direction.

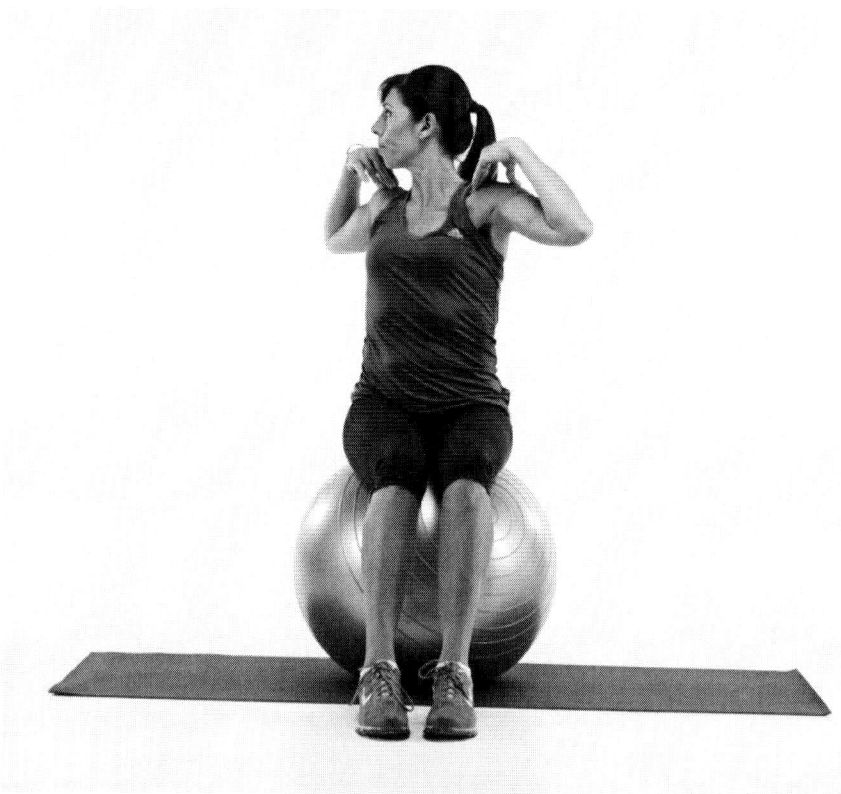

Key Points for Osteoporosis Exercises and Prolapse

- ♀ Osteoporosis is a condition where bones become brittle and prone to fracture.
- ♀ Osteoporosis can impact upon the pelvic floor.
- ♀ Women with osteoporosis are at increased risk of pelvic organ prolapse.
- ♀ Exercise is an important factor in the prevention and management of osteoporosis.
- ♀ Exercises known to most effectively promote increased bone density are high impact weight bearing exercises and high force strength training exercises.
- ♀ High impact exercises and high force resistance exercises can overload the pelvic floor and are inappropriate for most women with prolapse-related problems.
- ♀ A complete osteoporosis exercise program includes exercises for posture, muscle strength, balance and fitness.
- ♀ Women with osteoporosis and pelvic organ prolapse can reduce their injury risk by avoiding high impact and high force resistance exercises in favour of low impact weight bearing exercises and appropriate low-moderate strength training exercises.

10 Weight Management Exercises and Prolapse

Managing your body weight is an important part of managing your prolapse and preventing recurrent prolapse after surgery. Women often feel concerned about their ability to control their body weight when diagnosed with a prolapse, particularly if this means changing their exercise program. The fear of high impact weight loss exercises impacting upon the pelvic floor and worsening prolapse symptoms is often well justified. Returning to weight management exercise after prolapse surgery can be particularly worrying for women, especially when they realise the importance of weight management for the prevention of recurrent prolapse.

Weight Management and Prolapse

Body fat can load the pelvic floor, especially when stored as excess visceral fat. Visceral fat is a type of fat that accumulates within the trunk, around the abdominal organs and fills the spaces between the organs and the trunk. Visceral fat is not the same as the abdominal fat that may sit under your skin in rolls around your waist. Visceral fat causes the belly to protrude and it is associated with a pot-belly or apple shaped appearance, so your waist measurement may actually reflect the load on your pelvic floor. This means that most women with prolapse will benefit from managing their body weight and avoiding weight gain as part of their overall prolapse management strategy. Weight management is important for women seeking to avoid prolapse surgery since body weight has been identified as a risk factor for prolapse surgery in women.[15]

Exercise for Prolapse and Weight Management

Most women with mild-moderate prolapse can exercise for weight management and weight loss. Appropriate weight management exercise with prolapse problems involves doing sufficient and appropriate weight loss exercise. Understanding how to exercise for weight management can help you avoid weight gain, decrease the load on your pelvic floor if you are overweight and benefit your general health and wellbeing.

Choosing Appropriate Weight Loss Exercises

The most appropriate weight loss exercises for women with prolapse issues are low impact, aerobic exercises. These are exercises performed continuously, using the large muscle groups of the body, while keeping at least one foot on the ground. Exercises that involve the large muscle groups, such as your thigh muscles, will help you burn more energy during exercise.

Low impact weight management exercises include:

- Cycling (outdoors or stationary cycle)
- Walking (outdoors or treadmill)
- Lap swimming
- Water walking
- Cross country skiing (flat surface)
- Low impact dancing
- Low impact aerobic exercise equipment - stair machine, elliptical machine
- Low impact land-based aerobic exercise classes*
- Low impact water aerobics classes*

*Some classes may include intense abdominal core strength exercises requiring modification.

Weight Control Exercise Guidelines

To manage your weight with exercise, you need to ensure that the amount of physical work you do during exercise is sufficient i.e. how much time you spend exercising and how intensely you exercise.

A. *Exercise to prevent weight gain*

To prevent weight gain healthy adults require:

- 30-50 minutes of exercise on 5 days of the week or 150-250 minutes/week
- Continuous moderate intensity exercise
- Equivalent to burning 1200-2000 Calories(kcal)/week.[16]

Moderate intensity exercise means exercising at a level that feels 'somewhat hard'. When exercising at a moderate intensity you should feel that your heart rate and breathing are increased, you start to sweat and still comfortably carry out a conversation during exercise. Exercising at moderate intensity is usually feasible with a pelvic organ prolapse using appropriate low impact forms of exercise.

B. *Exercise to lose weight*

A dose-response relationship exists for physical activity and weight loss. This means that the more exercise you do, the more weight you can expect to lose.

For moderate weight loss of approximately 5-7.5kg, healthy adults need:

- 45 minutes-1.5 hours of exercise on 5 days of the week or 225-420 minutes/week
- Continuous moderate intensity exercise

Greater than 250 minutes/week of exercise will result in clinically significant weight loss, while less than 150 minutes/week results in minimal weight loss.[16]

Exercise to Reduce Abdominal Fat

To lose visceral (abdominal) fat and reduce the load on your pelvic floor, the more moderate intensity, low impact exercise you can do, the more weight you can expect to lose. Research shows that the more moderate intensity exercise healthy adults perform, the more abdominal fat they lose.[17] Varying the intensity of your exercise can reduce the amount of time you need to spend exercising and increase the amount of abdominal body fat you lose. Appropriate exercise intensity for reducing abdominal fat is outlined next.

Exercise Intensity for Weight Loss

If you have or are at risk of general health problems, or if you are obese, the most appropriate exercise intensity to commence with is low intensity. Low intensity exercise feels 'easy' and doesn't cause you to sweat or noticeably increase your breathing rate. If you are obese, your exercise program for fat loss will usually involve a gradual increase in the duration and frequency of your exercise sessions. If you are very overweight or obese, seek the guidance of an accredited exercise physiologist.

Moderate intensity exercise

Moderate intensity exercise is appropriate for weight loss in healthy adults.[16] Ideally, to achieve moderate (5-7.5kg) weight loss, moderate intensity exercise should be performed for at least 250 minutes/week. The combination of moderate intensity exercise combined with a moderate reduction in your energy intake will help you optimise your weight loss at this level of exercise intensity.

High intensity exercise

High intensity exercise is the most effective body weight and abdominal fat loss exercise for women who are able to perform this exercise intensity. High intensity exercise feels 'hard', makes you sweat and causes rapid deep breathing making it difficult to speak other than in short phrases.

Alternating high and low intensity exercise is a highly effective form of weight loss exercise. The LifeSprints[19] exercise program is a high and low intensity exercise program developed by researchers at the Medical Faculty University of NSW following their research into most effective weight loss exercise. LifeSprints is a 20-minute workout with 8 seconds of high intensity sprint exercise, followed by 12 seconds of easy exercise, 3 times a week. Research has shown that overweight women lost significantly more body fat (including abdominal fat) with short sessions of high intensity stationary cycling, than with longer moderate intensity sessions.[18] The women in this study exercised 3 times a week and maintained their normal diets during the 3 month study duration.

The LifeSprints exercise program has been used with a range of pelvic floor safe exercises including cycling, walking and stair walking and therefore provides an appropriate weight loss exercise alternative for some women with prolapse, without coexisting health problems that may prevent them from high intensity exercise.

High intensity exercise is not appropriate for all women. Consult with your doctor if you have any health risks (e.g. medications) or general health problems before commencing high intensity exercise.

Exercise and Diet for Weight Loss

If you don't have the time to do extended exercise sessions for weight loss, you can improve your weight loss results through appropriate diet - and this doesn't mean severely limiting how much energy you consume. The most effective diet and exercise combination for weight loss involves a moderate restriction in diet. Moderate diet and physical activity result in greater weight loss than diet alone.[16] Moderate dietary restriction is considered to be a reduction in energy intake of approximately 500-700 Calories (kcal)/day. Severe dietary restrictions in the range of 600-1000 Calories (kcal)/day combined with exercise do not increase overall weight loss.[16] If you are overweight or obese, seek the advice of a registered dietician for appropriate dietary guidelines.

Key Points for Weight Management Exercises and Prolapse

- Weight management is important for prolapse management.
- Excess body fat has the potential to load the pelvic floor, particularly when stored as excess visceral (abdominal) fat.
- Appropriate weight management exercise with a prolapse involves doing sufficient and appropriate weight loss exercise.
- The most appropriate weight loss exercises for women with prolapse are low impact aerobic exercises.
- To prevent weight gain, healthy adults need 30-50 minutes of continuous moderate intensity exercise on 5 days of the week or 150-250 minutes/week.
- For moderate weight loss (5-7.5kg) healthy adults need 45 minutes - 1.5 hours of continuous moderate intensity exercise on 5 days of the week or 225-420 minutes/week.
- The more moderate intensity exercise healthy adults perform the more abdominal fat they lose.
- The most effective diet and exercise combination for weight loss involves a moderate not severe restriction in diet.
- If you have or are at risk of general health problems, or if you are obese, the most appropriate exercise intensity to commence with is low intensity.
- Moderate intensity exercise is an appropriate exercise intensity for weight loss in adults.
- High intensity exercise is an effective body weight and abdominal fat loss exercise option for some women.
- Intermittent high intensity, low impact exercises are an effective and time efficient weight loss option for some women with pelvic floor problems.

References

[1] Bump R, Mattiasson A, Bo K, Brubaker L, DeLancey J, Klarskov P, Shull B, Smith A (1996) The standardization of terminology of female pelvic organ prolapse and pelvic floor dysfunction. *American Journal of Obstetrics & Gynecology,* 175:13.

[2] DeLancey J, Morgan D, Fenner D, Kearney R, Guire K, Miller JM, Hussain H, Umek W, Hsu Y, Ashton-Miller J (2007) Comparison of levator ani muscle defects and function in women with and without pelvic organ prolapse. *Obstetrics & Gynecology*, Feb;109(2 Pt 1):295-302.

[3] Brækken I, Majida M, Engh M, Bø K (2010) Can pelvic floor muscle training reverse pelvic organ prolapse and reduce prolapse symptoms? An assessor-blinded, randomized, controlled trial. *American Journal of Obstetrics and Gynecology,* 203(2):170e1-7.

[4] Hagen S, Stark D, Glazener C, Sinclair L, Ramsay I (2009) A randomised controlled trial of pelvic floor muscle training for stages I and II pelvic organ prolapse. *International Urogynecology Journal,* 20:45-51.

[5] Bo K and Frawley H (2007) Pelvic floor muscle training in prevention and treatment of POP. In: Bo K, Berghmans B, Morkved S, Van Kampen M (Eds). Evidence-based physical therapy for the pelvic floor. Philadelphia: Butterworth Heinemann Elsevier pp. 240-248.

[6] Balmforth J and Robinson D (2007) Pelvic organ prolapse. In: Bo K, Berghmans B, Morkved S, Van Kampen M (Eds). Evidence-based physical therapy for the pelvic floor. Philadelphia: Butterworth Heinemann Elsevier pp. 233-240.

[7] Bo K and Aschehoug A (2007) Strength training. In: Bo K, Berghmans B, Morkved S and Van Kampen M (Eds). Evidence-based physical therapy for the pelvic floor. Philadelphia: Butterworth Heinemann Elsevier pp.119-132.

[8] Michelle Kenway (2012) Pelvic Exercises Inside Out Strength DVD. Brisbane: Healthy Fit Solutions Pty Ltd.
https://www.pelvicexercises.com.au

[9] Michelle Kenway (2009) Inside Out - A complete guide to pelvic floor safe exercises for women. Brisbane: Sunset Digital Publications https://www.pelvicexercises.com.au

[10] American College of Sports Medicine (2011) Position stand. Quantity and quality of exercise for developing and maintaining cardiorespiratory, musculoskeletal, and neuromotor fitness in apparently healthy adults: guidance for prescribing exercise. *Medicine & Science in Sports & Exercise*, Jul;43(7):1334-59.

[11] Thompson J, O'Sullivan P, Briffa N and Neumann P (2007) Comparison of transperineal and transabdominal ultrasound in the assessment of voluntary pelvic floor muscle contractions and functional manoeuvres in continent and incontinent women. *International Urogynecology Journal*, Jul;18(7):779-86.

[12] Chiarelli P and Sibbritt D (2012) Osteoporosis and pelvic organ prolapse in Australian women: a longitudinal analysis. *International Urogynecology Journal*, Sept;23(2):s151-s152.

[13] Berecki-Gisolf J, Spallek M, Hockey R and Dobson A (2010) Height loss in elderly women is preceded by osteoporosis and is associated with digestive problems and urinary incontinence. *Osteoporosis International*, 21(3),479-485.

[14] Lanyon L (1996) Using functional loading to influence bone mass and architecture: objectives, mechanisms, and relationship with estrogen of the mechanically adaptive process in bone. *Bone*, Jan;18(1): S37-S43.

15 Mant J, Painter R, Vessey M (1997) Epidemiology of genital prolapse: observations from the Oxford Family Planning Association study. *BJOG: An International Journal of Obstetrics & Gynaecology*, 104(5):579-585.

[16] American College of Sports Medicine (2009) Position stand. Appropriate physical activity intervention strategies for weight loss and prevention of weight regain for adults. *Medicine & Science in Sports & Exercise*, Feb;41(2):459-471.

[17] Ohkawara K, Tanaka S, Miyachi M, Ishikawa-Takata K, Tabata I (2007) A dose-response relation between aerobic exercise and visceral fat reduction: systematic review of clinical trials. *International Journal of Obesity*, Dec;31(12):1786-1797.

[18] Trapp E, Chisholm D, Freund J, Boutcher S (2008) The effects of high-intensity intermittent exercise training on fat loss and fasting insulin levels of young women. *International Journal of Obesity*, 32(4), 684-691.

[19] Life Sprints http://www.lifesprints.com/home.html

My Journey to Pelvic Floor Safe Exercise

Exercise is an integral part of who I am and what I do - it has in many ways shaped the course of my life. As a schoolgirl and during my teenage years I was involved in netball, athletics, triathlon and gym-based exercise.

My personal interest in pelvic floor safe exercise emerged soon after the birth of my first baby. He was a big baby boy delivered by emergency forceps. Before his birth I had taken my pelvic floor for granted and it came as a shock to find that my pelvic floor and ability to exercise had changed. I was desperate to return to exercise after pregnancy and so my own pelvic floor journey began.

During my undergraduate Physiotherapy studies I recall only one lecture on women's health, so I had little idea about how to recover my pelvic floor and exercise safely. In the following years I returned to University and completed post graduate Physiotherapy studies, in Exercise for Women and Continence and Women's Health.

I have been fortunate to be able to put this knowledge into practice on a personal level and with my hospital-based gynaecology and private practice. Working with Urogynaecologists performing prolapse surgery made me concerned at the lack of information available to patients returning to exercise following childbirth and after prolapse surgery, and so the *Inside Out* program was born.

After writing my first book *Inside Out* I received thousands of emails from women worldwide - the lack of pelvic floor safe exercise and prolapse recovery information is indeed a global concern. Many women feel isolated and hopeless having little or no access to pelvic floor treatment and prolapse recovery information.

My hope is that by sharing my experiences and knowledge I can help you on your journey, so that you can enjoy exercise for your health and well being, feel confident in your body and enjoy your life to the fullest.

Michelle

Take the Prolapse Quiz

(1) Check your Individual Risk of Prolapse

Check the following prolapse risk factors that apply to you:

- □ Weak pelvic floor muscles
- □ Vaginal delivery
- □ Given birth two or more times
- □ Heavy lifting occupation
- □ Straining with constipation
- □ Chronic coughing
- □ Overweight (BMI greater than 25)
- □ Joint hypermobility (flexibility)
- □ Previous pelvic surgery (prolapse, continence, hysterectomy)
- □ Menopause
- □ Ageing

If you ticked one or more items, your risk of prolapse is increased.

(2) Check your Exercise Risks with Prolapse

Check the general exercise risks for prolapse that apply to you:

- □ Regular heavy lifting exercises
- □ Heavily loaded resistance exercises
- □ Repetitive high impact exercises
- □ Intense core abdominal exercises

Prolapse management involves addressing those individual risk factors under your control and modifying your exercise risks for prolapse by adhering to the pelvic floor safe exercise principles outlined in this book.

Other resources by Michelle Kenway

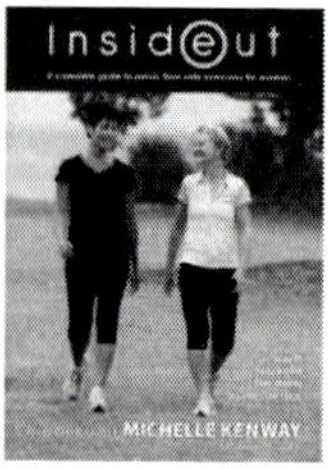

"Inside Out - A complete guide to pelvic floor safe exercises for women" (2009), Brisbane: Sunset Digital Publications.

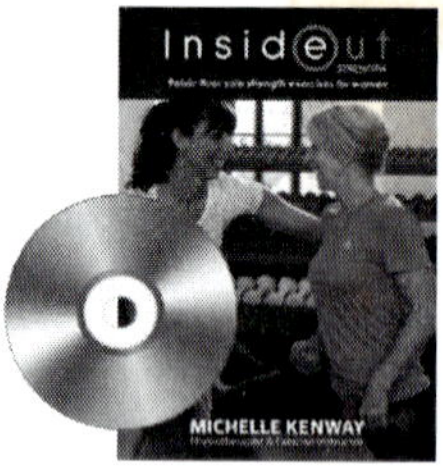

"Pelvic Exercises - Inside Out Strength" DVD (2012), Healthy Fit Solutions Pty Ltd.

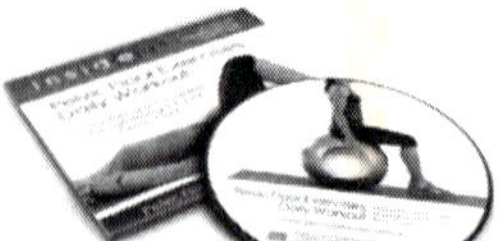

"Pelvic Floor Exercises Daily Workout" Physiotherapist-Guided Strengthening for your Pelvic Floor (CD), Healthy Fit Solutions Pty Ltd.

available at:

https://www.pelvicexercises.com.au